HEALTHY EASY PALEO RECIPES FOR ALL FAMILY

HEALTHY AND AMAZING RECIPES THAT UNLOCK THE FULL POTENTIAL OF YOUR VITAMIX, BLENDTEC, NINJA, OR OTHER HIGH-SPEED, HIGH-POWER BLENDER

MELISSA WALTRIP

COPYRIGHT

CONTENTS

SOUP RECIPES

JUICE RECIPES

SOUP RECIPES

ZUCCHINI AND BROCCOLI SOUP

INGREDIENTS

- 1 tbs olive oil
- 1 leek, pale section only, thickly sliced
- 1 garlic clove, crushed
- 1 zucchini, ends trimmed, coarsely chopped
- 1 head broccoli, florets and stems coarsely chopped
- 1 brushed potato, peeled, coarsely chopped
- 4 cups (1L) chicken or vegetable stock
- 1 cup (120g) frozen peas
- 1/2 cup (125ml) thickened cream
- Zucchini noodles, to serve
- Flat-leaf parsley leaves, to serve
- Chopped chives, to serve

METHOD

Step 1: Heat the oil in a large saucepan over medium heat. Add the leek and garlic and cook, stirring, for 5 mins or until leek softens. Add the zucchini, broccoli, potato and stock and bring to the boil. Reduce heat to medium-low and simmer, stirring occasionally, for 15 mins or until broccoli stems are very tender.

Step 2: Add the peas and cream and cook for 2 mins or until heated through. Remove from heat. Cool slightly. Use a stick blender to blend until smooth. Season. 3. Divide the soup among serving bowls. Top with zucchini noodles. Sprinkle with parsley and chives and serve immediately.

CAULIFLOWER SOUP WITH SMOKED CHEDDAR

INGREDIENTS

- 20g butter
- 2 tbs olive oil
- 1 brown onion, coarsely chopped
- 1 garlic clove, crushed
- 1 medium cauliflower, coarsely chopped
- 4 cups (1L) salt-reduced vegetable or chicken stock
- 1 cup (120g) coarsely grated smoked cheddar
- 1/2 cup (125ml) pouring (pure) cream or thickened cream
- 1 cup small cauliflower florets, extra
- 1/2 cup basil sprigs
- SMOKED ALMOND PESTO
- 60g pkt Coles Australian Baby Rocket
- 1/2 cup basil leaves
- 1/4 cup (20g) finely grated parmesan
- 1/3 cup (55g) smoked almonds, chopped
- 1 garlic clove, crushed
- 1/3 cup (80ml) avocado oil or olive oil

METHOD

Step 1: Heat the butter and half the oil in a large saucepan over medium heat. Add the onion and garlic and cook, stirring, for 5 mins or until onion softens. Add the cauliflower and stock. Increase heat to high and bring to the boil. Reduce heat to medium-low. Cook, stirring occasionally, for 15 mins or until the cauliflower is very tender. Remove from heat. Set aside to cool slightly.

Step 2: To make the smoked almond pesto, place rocket, basil, parmesan, almond and garlic in a food processor and process until finely chopped. With the motor running, add oil in a thin, steady stream until well combined. Season.

Step 3: Use a stick blender to carefully blend the cauliflower mixture in pan until very smooth. Add cheddar and cream. Stir until the cheddar melts. Place over low heat. Cook for 1-2 mins or until heated through. Season.

Step 4: Heat the remaining oil in a frying pan over high heat. Add the extra cauliflower and cook for 2-3 mins each side or until golden brown.

Step 5: Divide soup among serving bowls. Drizzle with the pesto. Top with fried cauliflower. Sprinkle with the basil.

PASTA SOUP WITH BEANS AND GREENS

INGREDIENTS

- 2 tbs extra virgin olive oil
- 100g sliced pancetta, finely chopped
- 1 brown onion, finely chopped
- 2 celery sticks, finely chopped
- 1 long red chilli, seeded, thinly sliced (optional)
- 4 garlic cloves, sliced
- 2 thyme sprigs
- 4 cups (1L) salt-reduced chicken stock
- 1 cup (260g) tomato passata
- 1 bunch Tuscan kale or green kale, trimmed, coarsely chopped
- 2 x 400g cans cannellini beans, rinsed, drained
- 3/4 cup (165g) risoni
- 40g-piece pecorino or parmesan
- Extra virgin olive oil, extra, to drizzle

METHOD

Step 1; Heat a large saucepan over medium-high heat. Add the oil and pancetta. Cook, stirring frequently, for 3 mins or until crisp. Using a slotted spoon, transfer pancetta to a plate. Add the onion, celery, chilli, if using, garlic and thyme to the pan. Season. Reduce heat to medium. Cook, stirring occasionally, for 12 mins or until the vegetables are tender.

Step 2: Add the stock, passata, kale, beans, 2 cups (500ml) water and 2 tsp salt. Cover and bring to a simmer. Cook for 5 mins or until the kale is tender. Add the risoni. Return to a simmer and cook, uncovered, stirring occasionally, for 8 mins or until the risoni is just tender. Season.

Step 3: Divide soup among serving bowls. Top with pancetta and finely grate over the pecorino or parmesan. Drizzle with extra oil and season with pepper.

HEARTY FRENCH CHICKEN SOUP

INGREDIENTS

- 1 tbsp extra virgin olive oil
- 4 chicken thigh fillets, trimmed
- 1 brown onion, halved, sliced
- 3 carrots, halved, thickly sliced diagonally
- 2 celery stalks, thickly sliced diagonally
- 3 garlic cloves, thinly sliced
- 1 dried bay leaf
- 3 sprigs fresh thyme
- 1/3 cup dry white wine
- 1 litre Massel Chicken Style Liquid Stock
- 500g potato, peeled, cut into chunks
- Roughly chopped fresh flat-leaf parsley leaves, to serve
- Toasted sliced baguette, to serve

METHOD

Step 1: Heat oil in a large saucepan over high heat. Season chicken with salt and pepper. Add chicken to pan. Cook for 4 minutes each side or until browned. Transfer to a plate.

Step 2: Add onion, carrot, celery, garlic, bay leaf and thyme to pan. Reduce heat to medium. Cook, stirring occasionally, for 6 minutes or until well browned. Add wine. Cook, scraping up brown bits from base of pan, for 1 minute. Return chicken to pan with stock and potato. Stir to combine. Bring to the boil. Reduce heat to medium. Simmer, covered, for 30 minutes or until vegetables are tender and chicken is cooked.

Step 3: Using tongs, transfer chicken to a board. Using 2 forks, roughly shred chicken. Remove and discard bay leaf and thyme.

Step 4: Return chicken to pan. Simmer for 2 minutes. Sprinkle with parsley. Serve with toasted sliced baguette.

CHICKEN POT PIE SOUP

INGREDIENTS

- 1 tbsp extra virgin olive oil
- 500g skinless chicken thigh fillets, trimmed, cut into 2cm pieces
- 3 middle bacon rashers, finely chopped
- 1 leek, white part only, sliced
- 1 garlic clove, crushed
- 2 tsp roughly chopped fresh rosemary leaves
- 2 tbsp cornflour
- 1 litre Massel salt reduced chicken style liquid stock
- 2/3 cup pure cream
- 2 cups frozen mixed vegetables (see note)
- 2 tbsp finely chopped fresh flat-leaf parsley leaves
- CHEESY PASTRY PUFFS
- 1/2 sheet frozen puff pastry, partially thawed
- 1 egg, lightly beaten
- 1/4 cup finely grated parmesan

METHOD

Step 1: Make Cheesy Pastry Puffs: Preheat oven to 220C/200C fan-forced. Line a baking tray with baking paper. Cut pastry into 5cm squares. Cut each square in half diagonally to form small triangles. Place pastry triangles on prepared tray. Brush with egg. Sprinkle with parmesan. Season with salt and pepper. Bake for 10 minutes or until golden and puffed.

Step 2: Meanwhile, heat the oil in a large heavy-based saucepan over medium-high heat. Cook chicken, in 2 batches, for 5 minutes or until browned all over. Transfer to a plate. Add bacon, leek, garlic and rosemary to pan. Cook, stirring, for 5 minutes or until leek has softened. Return chicken to pan.

Step 3: Blend cornflour with 1/4 cup stock in a large bowl. Stir in remaining stock. Add stock mixture to pan. Bring to the boil. Reduce heat to medium-low. Simmer for 5 minutes or until chicken is cooked through. Add cream and vegetables. Simmer for 3 minutes or until heated through. Season with salt and pepper.

Step 4: Ladle soup into bowls. Sprinkle with chopped parsley and serve with cheesy pastry puffs.

JAPANESE PUMPKIN SOUP

INGREDIENTS

- 1 tablespoon vegetable oil
- 1 brown onion, chopped
- 2cm piece fresh ginger, peeled, finely grated
- 2 garlic cloves, crushed
- 800g Jap pumpkin, peeled, cut into 3cm pieces
- 270ml can coconut milk
- 2 tablespoons white miso paste
- 3 cups salt-reduced vegetable stock
- 1 tablespoon tamari
- 1/4 cup fresh coriander sprigs
- 1 teaspoon shichimi togarashi (Japanese 7-spice blend)

METHOD

Step 1: Heat oil in a large saucepan over medium heat. Add onion.

Cook, stirring occasionally, for 3 to 4 minutes or until softened. Add ginger, garlic and pumpkin. Cook for 2 minutes.

Step 2: Reserve 1/3 cup coconut milk. Add miso, stock, tamari and remaining coconut milk to pan. Bring to the boil. Reduce heat to low. Simmer, covered, for 30 minutes or until pumpkin is tender.

Step 3: Remove from heat. Using a stick blender, blend until smooth. Season with salt and pepper. Ladle into bowls. Drizzle with reserved coconut milk and sprinkle with coriander and schichimi togarashi. Serve.

HAINANESE CHICKEN AND RICE SOUP

INGREDIENTS

- 1.6kg Coles RSPCA Approved Australian Whole Chicken
- 4 spring onions, cut into 5cm lengths
- 5cm-piece ginger, thickly sliced
- 2 garlic cloves, crushed
- 1/3 cup (80ml) light soy sauce
- 1/3 cup (80ml) Chinese cooking wine
- 2 tsp sesame oil
- 1/3 cup (65g) jasmine rice
- 1 bunch baby buk choy, sliced lengthways
- 1 bunch baby choy sum, cut into 5cm lengths
- 5cm-piece ginger, extra, peeled, cut into matchsticks

METHOD

Step 1: Place chicken, spring onion, ginger, garlic, soy sauce, Chinese cooking wine and half the oil in a large saucepan. Add enough cold water to the pan to cover chicken. Place over high heat and bring to the boil. Reduce heat to low. Cook, uncovered, skimming foam from surface occasionally, for 2 hours or until the chicken is cooked through and meat is falling off the bone.

Step 2: Use tongs to transfer the chicken to a heatproof bowl. Set aside to cool slightly. Use 2 forks to shred the meat, discarding the skin and bones.

Step 3: Meanwhile, strain the cooking liquid through a sieve into a clean saucepan. Discard solids. Place over medium heat. Add the rice. Cook for 15 mins or until rice is tender. Return the chicken to the pan with the buk choy, choy sum, extra ginger and the remaining oil. Season.

Step 4: Divide the soup evenly among serving bowls.

MISO CHICKEN NOODLE SOUP

INGREDIENTS

- 200g dried noodles of choice (see notes)
- 20g fresh ginger
- 1000g Massel Chicken Style Liquid Stock
- 50g shiro (white) miso paste
- 40g tamari
- 500g chicken tenderloins, cut into halves
- 200-300g savoy cabbage leaves, cut into thin slices
- 1 bunch Asian greens of choice, cut into pieces (2 cm)
- 8 fresh shiitake mushrooms, finely sliced
- 100g fresh enoki mushrooms
- Toasted sesame seeds, for sprinkling
- 3 spring onions, trimmed and cut into thin slices

METHOD

Step 1: Prepare noodles as per packet instructions.

Step 2: Place ginger into mixing bowl and chop 3 sec/speed 7.

Step 3: Add stock, miso and tamari and heat 10 min/100C/speed 1.

Step 4: Add the chicken and gently poach 8-10 min/90C or until cooked. Using a slotted spoon remove the chicken from the soup and place in a thermal serving bowl (ThermoServer®) and cover to keep warm. Leave soup in the mixing bowl.

Step 5: Place Varoma into position and weigh cabbage into it, then add the greens. Secure Varoma lid and cook 5-8 min/Varoma/speed 2 or until just cooked. Meanwhile, shred the reserved chicken and divide the noodles between 4 serving bowls, then top with the shredded chicken. Remove the Varoma and divide cooked cabbage and greens between the serving bowls.

Step 6: Add mushrooms and cook 2 min/100C/speed 1. Divide soup and mushrooms between the serving bowls. Top with spring onions/ shallots and sprinkle with toasted sesame seeds.

ULTIMATE QUARANTINE SOUP

INGREDIENTS

- 2 tablespoons extra virgin olive oil
- 1 brown onion, finely chopped
- 3 garlic cloves, finely chopped
- 1 tablespoon chopped fresh ginger
- 2 teaspoons ground turmeric, plus extra to sprinkle (optional)
- 1 teaspoon cumin seeds, crushed
- Pinch dried chilli flakes, plus extra to sprinkle (optional)
- 400g can tomato polpi or crushed tomatoes
- 3 tsp vegetable or chicken stock powder
- 4 dried bay leaves
- 400g can lentils, drained, rinsed
- 400g can chickpeas, drained, rinsed
- 150g frozen spinach
- Juice of half a lemon, plus extra wedges to serve
- Greek yoghurt, to dollop

METHOD

Step 1: Heat the oil in a large saucepan over high heat. Add the onion. Reduce heat to low and cook, stirring occasionally, for 5 minutes or until softened. Add the garlic and ginger and cook, stirring, for 1 minute or until aromatic. Add the turmeric, cumin and chilli and stir to coat.

Step 2: Add the tomato to the saucepan. Fill the empty tomato can with water and add to the saucepan. Add another can of water. Stir in the stock powder and bay leaves. Increase heat to high and bring to the boil. Reduce heat to low and simmer, uncovered for 15 minutes. Stir through the lentils and chickpeas. Simmer for a further 20 minutes or until thickened.

Step 3: Add the spinach and cook, stirring occasionally,for 5-10 minutes or until spinach has thawed. Add the lemon juice and season.

Step 4: Divide among serving bowls and serve with yoghurt and extra turmeric and chilli if desired.

EXPRESS WONTON NOODLE SOUP

INGREDIENTS

- 5 garlic cloves, peeled
- 5 garlic cloves, peeled 4cm piece ginger, peeled, coarsely chopped
- 1 teaspoon whole black peppercorns
- 2 tablespoons vegetable oil
- 700g (4) boneless chicken thigh fillets
- 2L (8 cups) Massel chicken style liquid stock
- 2 whole star anise
- 80ml (1/3 cup) soy sauce
- 12 frozen wontons or dumplings
- 400g cooked Chinese-style egg noodles (such as shelf-ready thin hokkien noodles or cooked fresh thin Chinese egg noodles)
- 4 baby pak choy, quartered lengthways
- Thinly sliced long fresh red chilli, to serve

METHOD

Step 1: Use a mortar and pestle or a small blender to combine the garlic, ginger and peppercorns into a rough paste.

Step 2: Heat the vegetable oil in a large saucepan over medium-high heat. Season the chicken with salt and cook 2-3 minutes each side or until just starting to colour. Add the garlic mixture and cook, stirring, for about a minute or until aromatic. Add the stock, star-anise and soy sauce. Bring to a gentle simmer then reduce heat to low and cook for 10 minutes or until chicken is cooked through.

Step 3: Meanwhile, fill another saucepan with water. Place over high heat. Once boiling, add wontons or dumplings. Cook for 3-4 minutes or until just cooked through. Drain.

Step 4: Divide the noodles and pak choy among serving bowls and top with the wontons or dumplings.

Step 5: Use tongs to transfer the cooked chicken from the soup to a chopping board. Slice the chicken and divide among bowls. Strain the soup and discard the solids. Season with salt or soy sauce, to taste. Ladle the hot soup into the bowls. Sprinkle with sliced red chilli to serve.

RECIPE NOTES

A variety of shelf-ready noodles are available in the Asian section of major supermarkets. Fresh thin Chinese egg noodles are sold in the fridge section of Asian supermarkets and some major supermarkets. Follow packet directions

FOR PREPARATION

Always cook the wontons or dumplings and noodles separately to the soup. Cooking them in the soup can affect

the flavour of the broth.

Slicing the pak choy helps it to cook when the hot soup is poured over. If you're using larger pak choy, buk choy or other green vegetables, blanch them in the boiling water before cooking the wontons or dumplings (in step 3).

GREEN PESTO VEGETABLE SOUP

INGREDIENTS

- 1 tbs olive oil
- 1 brown onion, finely chopped
- 1 brushed potato, peeled, finely chopped
- 2 garlic cloves, crushed
- 3 zucchini, finely chopped
- 4 cups (1L) vegetable or chicken stock
- 100g farfalle pasta
- 2 cups (240g) frozen peas
- 1/2 cup (125ml) thickened cream
- GREEN PESTO
- ½ cup basil leaves
- 60g pkt Coles Australian Baby Rocket
- 2 garlic cloves
- 1/4 cup (40g) pine nuts, toasted
- 1 tbs pepitas (pumpkin seeds), toasted
- 1/3 cup (25g) finely grated parmesan
- 1/3 cup (80ml) olive oil

METHOD

Step 1: Heat the oil in a large saucepan over medium heat. Add the onion, potato and garlic and cook, stirring, for 5 mins or until onion softens. Add the zucchini and cook for 2 mins or until tender. Add the stock and increase heat to high. Bring to the boil. Reduce heat to medium and cook for 10 mins or until the potato and zucchini are tender.

Step 2: Meanwhile, to make the green pesto, place basil, rocket, garlic, pine nuts, pepitas and parmesan in a food processor. Process until finely chopped. With the motor running, add oil in a thin, steady stream until combined. Season.

Step 3: Cook the pasta in a small saucepan of boiling water for 10 mins or until al dente. Add ½ cup (60g) peas. Cook for 1 min. Drain well. Transfer to a bowl with 1 tbs of pesto and toss to combine.

Step 4: Add the remaining peas to the soup. Cook for 5 mins or until heated through. Stir in the cream. Remove from heat. Set aside to cool slightly. Use a stick blender to blend until smooth. Add half the remaining pesto. Stir to combine.

Step 5: Divide the soup among serving bowls. Drizzle with the remaining pesto. Top with the pasta mixture.

RECIPE NOTES

SERVE WITH shaved parmesan, basil leaves, toasted pepitas and extra virgin olive oil.

HEARTY VEGETABLE AND LENTIL SOUP

INGREDIENTS

- 1 brown onion, finely chopped
- 3 cups (420g) frozen mixed vegetables

- 400g can lentils, rinsed, drained
- 400g can diced tomatoes
- 2 cups (500ml) salt-reduced vegetable stock

METHOD

Step 1: Heat a large non-stick saucepan over medium heat. Add the onion and 1 tbs water and cook, stirring, for 3 mins or until the onion softens.

Step 2: Add the vegetables, lentils, tomato, stock and 4 cups (1L) water to the pan. Bring to the boil. Reduce heat to low and bring to a simmer. Cook for 10 mins or until vegetables are tender and the mixture is heated through.

RECIPE NOTES

SWAP ME: You can use any frozen vegetables in this soup, such as cauliflower or broccoli florets.

RATATOUILLE SOUP WITH CHEESE TORTELLINI

INGREDIENTS

- 2 tbs olive oil
- 1 brown onion, finely chopped
- 2 garlic cloves, crushed
- 1 eggplant, coarsely chopped
- 2 tsp dried Italian herbs
- 1 tbs tomato paste
- 3 cups (750ml) vegetable stock
- 1 tbs red wine vinegar
- 1 tbs brown sugar
- 4 vine-ripened cherry tomatoes, coarsely chopped
- 285g jar whole piquillo peppers, drained, coarsely chopped
- 200g cheese tortellini
- 2 zucchini, thinly sliced
- 2 cups (60g) Tuscan kale or green kale, trimmed, leaves chopped
- 1/3 cup (90g) Coles Basil Pesto

EQUIPMENT

slow cooker

METHOD

Step 1: Heat the oil in a large frying pan over medium-high heat. Add the onion, garlic and eggplant, Cook, stirring, for 4 mins or until tender. Transfer to a slow cooker.

Step 2: Add the herbs, tomato paste, stock, vinegar, sugar, tomato and peppers to the slow cooker. Season. Cover and cook for 2 hours on high (or 4 hours on low) or until the vegetables are tender.

Step 3: Add the tortellini. Cook, covered, for 20 mins. Add the zucchini and kale and stir until combined and heated through.

Step 4: Divide the soup among serving bowls. Top with pesto to serve.

CREAMY TORTELLINI MINESTRONE SOUP

INGREDIENTS

- 2 celery sticks, finely chopped
- 2 tablespoons olive oil
- 100g pancetta, coarsely chopped
- 2 carrots, peeled, finely chopped
- 1 brown onion, finely chopped
- 2 celery sticks, finely chopped
- 2 garlic cloves, crushed
- 1litre (4 cups) Massel Chicken Style Liquid Stock
- 400g can diced Italian tomatoes
- 325g pkt spinach and ricotta tortellini
- 400g can borlotti beans, rinsed, drained
- 80g (2/3 cup) crème fraîche
- 75g (1/4 cup) bought basil pesto
- Fresh small basil leaves, to serve

METHOD

Step 1: Heat oil in a stockpot over medium-high heat. Add the pancetta, carrot, celery and onion. Cook, stirring often, for 5-8 minutes or until soft. Add the garlic and cook, stirring, for 30 seconds or until aromatic.

Step 2: Add the stock and tomatoes. Bring to the boil. Add the tortellini and borlotti beans. Cover and bring back to a gentle simmer. Uncover and reduce the heat to medium. Cook, stirring often, for 2-3 minutes or until the tortellini is al dente.

Step 3: Meanwhile, combine the crème fraîche and 2 tbs pesto in a bowl until well combined.

Step 4: Ladle the minestrone among serving bowls. Top with a dollop of the pesto cream and the remaining pesto. Sprinkle with basil to serve.

RECIPE NOTES

- If pancetta isn't available, replace with bacon.
- Don't like tortellini? Use ravioli instead or replace with small dried pasta, such as macaroni, and cook for 10-12 minutes or until al dente.

MEXICAN-STYLE SEAFOOD SOUP

INGREDIENTS

- 1 tbs olive oil
- 1 brown onion, finely chopped
- 1 large carrot, peeled, finely chopped
- 2 celery sticks, finely chopped
- 300g can corn kernels, drained
- 200g jar taco sauce
- 4 cups (1L) Salt Reduced Chicken Stock
- 500g thawed seafood marinara mix (from the deli)
- 1 small avocado, stoned, peeled, finely chopped

METHOD

Step 1: Heat the oil in a large saucepan over medium heat. Add the onion, carrot and celery and cook, stirring occasionally, for 10 mins or until the onion softens.

Step 2: Add the corn, taco sauce and stock and bring to the boil. Cover and cook for 5 mins or until the vegetables are tender. Add the marinara mix and cook, uncovered, for 3 mins or until the seafood changes colour and is just cooked through.

Step 3: Divide the soup evenly among serving bowls. Top with avocado. Season to serve.

RECIPE NOTES

Serve with coriander sprigs and lime wedges.

CRUNCH TIME: For a touch of crunch, top the soup with broken corn chips or tortilla chips just before serving.

CHICKEN, BACON AND VERMICELLI SOUP

INGREDIENTS

- 2 tablespoons olive oil
- 200g bought diced bacon
- 1 brown onion, finely chopped
- 500g chicken breast fillets, cut into 2cm pieces
- 140g (1/2 cup) tomato paste
- 400g can cannellini beans, rinsed, drained
- 400g can creamed corn
- 10 fresh thyme sprigs, plus extra to serve
- 1L (4 cups) chicken stock
- 125g dried vermicelli pasta
- Finely grated parmesan, to serve

METHOD

Step 1: Heat 1 tbs olive oil in a large saucepan over high heat. Add the bacon and cook, stirring, for 3-4 minutes or until crispy. Transfer the bacon to a plate.

Step 2: Heat the remaining oil in the pan over medium-high heat. Add the onion and chicken to the pan and cook, stirring, for 6 minutes or until golden and cooked through. Add the tomato paste, beans, corn, thyme and stock. Season. Cover. Bring to the boil.

Step 3: Add the pasta to the chicken mixture and cook for 6 minutes or until the pasta is al dente. Divide the soup among serving bowls. Top with bacon, extra thyme and parmesan to serve.

RECIPE NOTES

To prep ahead: Make the soup up to the end of step 2. Place in an airtight container and freeze for up to 3 months. To serve, reheat and continue cooking from step 3.

CREAMY MUSHROOM SOUP

INGREDIENTS

- 1 large brown onion, diced
- Olive or vegetable oil
- 6 large big potatoes, peeled and cut into small pieces
- 1/2 teaspoon caraway seeds, ground
- 3 large bay leaves
- Whole mushrooms (230 g in jar), sliced
- 500 g fresh button mushrooms button, peeled then sliced
- 1 heap tbsp of fresh dill, chopped
- 300 ml thickened cream
- Vegeta gourmet stock seasoning
- 4 boiled eggs
- Salt
- Black pepper
- 2 tbsp cornflour mixed with a little water

METHOD

Step 1: Heat little oil in a large saucepan over medium heat. Add onion and cook until translucent.

Step 2: Add caraway seeds stir then add potatoes, bay leaves and slowly pour in about 2L boiling water.

Step 3: Cover with lid and simmer until the potatoes start soften then add both mushrooms. Cook until the mushrooms are soft.

Step 4: Pick out the bay leaves. Add thickened cream, dill and slowly pour in cornflour mixed with little water. Keep stirring and cook until bubbling and the soup thickens.

Step 5; Taste and season with Vegeta, salt and pepper.

Step 6: Serve on a plate and top with halved cooked egg.

BEEF MASSAMAN SOUP

INGREDIENTS

- 2 tbsp rice bran oil
- 500g gravy beef, fat trimmed, cut into 3cm pieces
- 1 brown onion, halved, thinly sliced
- 1/3 cup massaman curry paste
- 1 litre Massel salt reduced chicken style liquid stock
- 2 dried bay leaves
- 1 cinnamon stick
- 2 large desiree potatoes, peeled, cut into 2cm pieces
- 300g sweet potato, peeled, cut into 2cm pieces
- 1/2 cup coconut milk, plus extra to serve
- 1 tbsp fish sauce
- 1 tbsp lime juice
- Unsalted roasted peanuts, to serve
- Fried shallots, to serve
- Fresh coriander leaves, to serve

METHOD

Step 1: Heat half the oil in a large heavy-based saucepan over medium-high heat. Cook beef, in 2 batches, for 5 to 6 minutes or until browned all over. Transfer to a bowl.

Step 2: Heat remaining oil in pan. Add onion. Cook, stirring, for 5 minutes. Add curry paste. Cook, stirring, for 1 minute. Return beef to pan. Stir to coat. Add stock, bay leaves and cinnamon. Cover. Bring to boil. Reduce heat to low. Simmer, stirring occasionally, for 1 hour 30 minutes. Add potato and sweet potato. Cook, covered, for 30 minutes or until beef and potato are tender.

Step 3: Discard bay leaves and cinnamon. Stir in coconut milk, fish sauce and lime juice. Ladle soup into bowls. Top with peanuts, fried shallots and coriander leaves, and drizzle with extra coconut milk to serve.

LEFTOVER LAMB SOUP

INGREDIENTS

- 120g dried vegeroni spiral pasta
- 1 tbsp extra virgin olive oil
- 1 brown onion, finely chopped
- 2 garlic cloves, crushed
- 1 carrot, diced
- 1 celery stalk, diced
- 1.5 litres vegetable liquid stock
- 1 cup fresh peas or frozen peas
- 100g sugar snap peas, trimmed
- 1 bunch baby asparagus, cut into 4cm lengths
- 1 1/2 cups cold shredded leftover cooked lamb (see notes)
- 2 tbsp fresh curly parsley, torn

METHOD

Step 1: Cook pasta following packet directions. Drain. Refresh under cold water.

Step 2: Meanwhile, heat oil in a large saucepan over medium-high heat. Add onion, garlic, carrot and celery. Cook, stirring occasionally, for 3 minutes or until vegetables have softened. Add stock. Bring to a simmer. Cover. Reduce heat to low. Cook for 15 minutes.

Step 3: Add peas, sugar snap peas, asparagus and lamb. Simmer for 2 minutes or until lamb is heated through. Remove from heat. Stir in pasta. Season with salt and pepper. Sprinkle soup with parsley. Serve.

COLCANNON POTATO AND PORK SOUP

INGREDIENTS

- 2 tbs olive oil
- 2 leeks, pale section only, thickly sliced
- 1 brown onion, finely chopped
- 2 garlic cloves, crushed
- 2 cups (160g) shredded green cabbage
- 1 large (about 1kg) Coles Australian Smoked Meaty Pork Leg Hock
- 3 Red Royale potatoes, peeled, chopped
- 2 bay leaves
- 4 cups (1L) chicken stock
- 3 spring onions, thinly sliced
- 1/4 cup (60ml) thickened cream

METHOD

Step 1: Heat half the oil in a large non-stick frying pan over medium heat. Add the leek, onion and garlic. Cook, stirring, for 4 mins or until onion softens. Transfer to a slow cooker. Add cabbage, pork hock, potato, bay leaves and stock. Cover and cook for 3 hours on high (or 5 hours on low) or until the potato and pork are tender. Turn off slow cooker.

Step 2: Transfer the pork hock to a heatproof bowl. Cool slightly. Use 2 forks to shred the meat, discarding the bone and rind. Heat the remaining oil in a non-stick frying pan over high heat. Cook the pork, in 2 batches, stirring, for 3-5 mins or until crisp. Transfer to a plate.

Step 3: Remove bay leaves from soup and discard. Use a stick blender to carefully blend soup until smooth. Divide among serving bowls. Season. Top with pork and spring onion. Drizzle with cream.

RECIPE NOTES

Allow for cooking time.

ON THE STOVE: Don't own a slow cooker? Cook soup in a casserole pan, partially covered, over low heat for 2 hours or until pork is tender.

TOMATO AND SWEET POTATO SOUP

INGREDIENTS

- 1 tbs olive oil
- 1 brown onion, coarsely chopped
- 2 celery sticks, coarsely chopped
- 2 garlic cloves, crushed
- 1kg gold sweet potato, peeled, cut into 2cm pieces
- 700g btl Leggo's Passata with Italian Herbs
- 4 cups (1L) vegetable or chicken stock
- 4 slices prosciutto
- 1/2 cup (120g) sour cream
- Oregano leaves, to serve
- Extra virgin olive oil, to drizzle
- Toasted baguette slices, to serve

METHOD

Step 1: Heat olive oil in a large saucepan over medium heat. Add the onion and celery and cook, stirring occasionally, for 5 mins or until onion softens. Add garlic. Cook, stirring, for 1 min or until aromatic.

Step 2: Stir in sweet potato, Leggo's Passata with Italian Herbs and stock. Cover. Bring to the boil over medium heat. Reduce heat to low. Simmer, covered, for 15-20 mins or until the sweet potato is soft. Remove from heat.

Step 3: Preheat grill on medium-high. Line a baking tray with foil. Spray with olive oil spray. Arrange the prosciutto on prepared tray. Spray with oil. Cook under the grill for 2 mins each side or until golden brown.

Step 4: Use a stick blender to carefully blend the soup until smooth (if it's too thick, add a little more stock or water). Divide among serving bowls. Tear prosciutto into large pieces. Top soup with sour cream, prosciutto and oregano. Drizzle with extra virgin olive oil. Season. Serve with the toast.

MOUSSAKA SOUP

INGREDIENTS

- 2 lamb shanks
- 1/3 cup extra virgin olive oil
- 1 brown onion, finely chopped
- 3 garlic cloves, thinly sliced
- 1 dried bay leaf
- 2 tbsp tomato paste
- 1/2 tsp ground allspice
- 1/2 tsp ground cinnamon
- 400g can diced tomatoes
- 2 cups Massel Chicken Style Liquid Stock
- 400g can chickpeas, drained, rinsed
- 1 tsp dried oregano
- 2 eggplants, partially peeled, cut into 1.5cm pieces
- Plain low-fat Greek-style yoghurt, to serve
- Shredded fresh mint leaves, to serve
- Chargrilled Lebanese bread, to serve

METHOD

Step 1: Season lamb with salt and pepper. Heat 1 tablespoon oil in a large saucepan over high heat. Add lamb. Cook, turning, for 8 minutes or until browned all over. Transfer to a plate.

Step 2: Reduce heat to medium. Add onion, garlic and bay leaf. Cook, stirring occasionally, for 5 minutes or until softened. Add tomato paste and spices. Cook, stirring, for 1 minute. Add tomatoes, stock, chickpeas, oregano and 2 cups water. Bring to the boil. Cover. Reduce heat to medium-low. Cook for 1 hour 40 minutes or until lamb is very tender.

Step 3: Meanwhile, heat 1 1/2 tablespoons remaining oil in a large frying pan over high heat. Add half the eggplant. Cook, stirring occasionally, for 10 minutes or until golden. Transfer to a plate. Repeat with remaining oil and eggplant.

Step 4: Using tongs, transfer lamb to a board. Using 2 forks, shred meat. Discard bones. Remove and discard bay leaf. Return shredded lamb to pan with eggplant. Simmer, covered, for 20 minutes. Divide soup among serving bowls. Dollop with yoghurt and sprinkle with mint. Serve with chargrilled Lebanese bread.

RECIPE NOTES

To partially peel the eggplant, peel 1 strip lengthways, leave a strip of skin, then peel another strip. Continue alternating peeling to make stripes.

PEA AND HAM SOUP

INGREDIENTS

- 2 tbs olive oil
- 1 brown onion, finely chopped
- 1 leek, pale section only, thinly sliced
- 1kg potatoes, peeled, finely chopped
- 4 cups (1L) Coles Real Salt Reduced Chicken Stock
- 3 cups (360g) frozen peas
- 350g thickly sliced ham, chopped
- 1/3 cup (80ml) thickened cream

METHOD

Step 1: Heat half the oil in a saucepan over medium heat. Add onion and leek. Cook, stirring, for 5 mins or until onion softens.

Step 2; Add the potato, stock and 2 cups (500ml) water. Bring to the boil. Reduce heat to low and simmer for 10 mins or until the potato is tender. Stir in the peas. Cook for 5 mins or until the peas are tender.

Step 3: Meanwhile, heat remaining oil in a frying pan over medium-high heat. Cook ham, stirring, for 5 mins or until golden. Transfer to a plate lined with paper towel.

Step 4: Transfer half the vegetable mixture to a heatproof bowl and reserve. Use a stick blender to carefully blend the remaining vegetable mixture in the pan until smooth. Stir in the reserved vegetable mixture. Divide the soup among serving bowls. Drizzle with cream and top with the ham. Season.

RECIPE NOTES

Serve with finely chopped chives and toasted Coles Bakery Stone Baked by Laurent White Sourdough Vienna.

QUICK TRICK: To save you time, we've used frozen peas in this soup instead of the traditional dried green split peas.

MEXICAN CHICKEN SOUP

INGREDIENTS

- 1 tbs olive oil
- 1 red onion, finely chopped
- 1 tbs taco seasoning
- 1 Coles RSPCA Approved Australian Chicken Breast Fillet
- 300g jar mild tomato salsa
- 4 cups (1L) chicken stock
- 1 corn cob, husk and silk removed
- 400g can black beans, rinsed, drained

METHOD

Step 1: Heat the oil in a large saucepan over medium heat. Add the onion and cook, stirring, for 5 mins or until onion softens. Add taco seasoning and cook, stirring, for 1 min or until aromatic.

Step 2: Add chicken, salsa and stock. Bring to a simmer. Cook, partially covered, for 15 mins or until chicken is cooked through. Use a slotted spoon to transfer chicken to a heatproof bowl. Set aside for 5 mins to cool slightly.

Step 3: Use a small serrated knife to cut down the side of the corn to remove the kernels. Use two forks to coarsely shred the chicken. Return the chicken to the soup with the corn kernels and beans. Cook for 5 mins or until heated through. Season.

BEEF STROGANOFF SOUP

INGREDIENTS

- 3 cups Massel Chicken Style Liquid Stock
- 1/2 x 20g packet dried porcini mushrooms
- 700g piece beef topside roast
- 1/3 cup extra virgin olive oil
- 2 brown onions, thinly sliced
- 3 sprigs fresh thyme
- 1 dried bay leaf
- 3 garlic cloves, finely chopped
- 250g button mushrooms, thickly sliced
- 250g fusilli avellinesi pasta (see notes)
- 1/2 cup thickened cream
- Roughly chopped fresh chives, to serve

METHOD

Step 1: Bring stock and 3 cups water to the boil in a medium saucepan over high heat. Add porcini. Set aside.

Step 2: Meanwhile, season beef with salt and pepper. Heat 1 tablespoon oil in a large saucepan over high heat. Add beef. Cook, turning, for 8 minutes or until well browned on all sides. Transfer to a plate. Carefully wipe pan clean with paper towel.

Step 3: Heat 2 tablespoons remaining oil in pan over high heat. Add onion, thyme and bay leaf. Season with salt and pepper. Cook, stirring occasionally, for 6 minutes or until softened. Reduce heat to medium. Add garlic. Cook for 4 minutes or until well browned. Strain stock mixture into pan with beef (see notes). Roughly chop porcini. Add to pan. Bring to the boil. Cover. Reduce heat to medium-low. Cook for 1 hour 30 minutes or until beef is tender.

Step 4: Meanwhile, heat remaining oil in a large frying pan over high heat. Add button mushrooms. Cook, stirring occasionally, for 5 minutes or until golden.

Step 5: Using tongs, transfer beef to a board. Using 2 forks, shred meat. Remove and discard herbs. Return beef to pan. Bring to the boil. Add button mushrooms and pasta. Boil, partially covered, for 15 minutes or until pasta is tender. Add cream. Stir to combine. Serve soup sprinkled with chives.

RECIPE NOTES

You can use any short pasta for this recipe.

To ensure beef cooks evenly, make sure it is immersed in stock mixture. If the roast is too big, simply cut it in half.

CREAMY MUSHROOM RISOTTO SOUP

INGREDIENTS

- 1.5 litres salt-reduced vegetable stock
- 2 fresh thyme sprigs, plus extra to serve
- 60g butter
- 200g Swiss brown mushrooms, sliced
- 200g button mushrooms, halved
- 150g packet pasta mushroom mix (see notes)
- 1 brown onion, finely chopped
- 1 garlic clove, crushed
- 1 1/2 cups arborio rice
- 1/3 cup Bulla Cooking Cream
- 1/2 cup finely grated parmesan, plus extra to serve

METHOD

Step 1: Place stock and thyme sprigs in a saucepan over medium-high heat. Cover. Bring to the boil. Reduce heat to low.

Step 2: Meanwhile, melt 40g butter in a large heavy-based saucepan over high heat. Add mushrooms. Cook, stirring occasionally, for 5 minutes or until well browned. Transfer to a bowl. Cover to keep warm.

Step 3: Melt remaining butter in same pan over medium-high heat. Cook onion, stirring, for 5 minutes or until softened. Add garlic. Cook for 1-minute or until fragrant. Add rice. Cook, stirring, for 1 minute or until rice is coated

Step 4: Reduce heat to low. Add 1/3 cup hot stock to rice. Cook, stirring, until liquid is absorbed. Repeat with stock, ⅓ cup at a time, allowing liquid to be absorbed before each addition, until rice is almost tender (see notes). Add remaining stock and half the mushrooms. Cook for 3 to 4 minutes or until rice is tender.

Step 5: Stir in cream and parmesan. Top with remaining mushrooms, extra parmesan and extra thyme. Serve.

RECIPE NOTES

- The pasta mushroom mix is available from Woolworths.
- For this process, you'll use about 3/4 of the stock and it will take about 35 to 40 minutes.
- Risotto soup will thicken on standing. Add more stock or water if needed.

CURRIED PUMPKIN SOUP WITH CHICKEN

INGREDIENTS

- 1 tbs peanut oil
- 500g pkt Coles Australian Diced Butternut Pumpkin
- 1/3 cup (100g) korma curry paste
- 3 cups (750ml) chicken stock
- 270ml coconut cream
- 1 cup (160g) shredded Coles RSPCA Approved Hot Roast Chicken Breast
- 100g green beans, trimmed, halved crossways
- 1/2 cup (140g) Greek-style yoghurt
- 1 long green chilli, sliced (optional)
- 1/4 cup (20g) Coles Shredded Coconut, toasted
- 2 tbs chopped chives

METHOD

Step 1: Heat the oil in a large saucepan over medium-high heat. Add the pumpkin and cook for 2 mins. Add curry paste. Cook for 30 secs or until fragrant.

Step 2: Add stock to the pan. Bring to the boil. Reduce heat to medium. Simmer for 5 mins or until pumpkin is tender. Remove from heat. Cool slightly. Use a stick blender to blend until smooth.

Step 3: Add coconut cream and place over medium heat. Bring to a simmer. Add chicken and beans. Cook for 2 mins or until beans are bright green and tender.

Step 4: Divide soup among serving bowls. Top with the yoghurt. Sprinkle with chilli, if using, coconut and chives.

RECIPE NOTES

Serve with buttered Coles Naan Bread, flat-leaf parsley leaves and chopped toasted cashews.

HEALTHY CHICKEN NOODLE SOUP

INGREDIENTS

- 100g dried rice vermicelli noodles
- 2 teaspoons macadamia oil
- 1 large brown onion, finely chopped
- 2 large celery sticks, finely chopped
- 2 garlic cloves, crushed
- 3cm piece fresh ginger, peeled, thinly sliced
- 1 long fresh red chilli, deseeded, finely chopped
- 1 stick lemongrass, cut into 4cm lengths, bruised
- 400g lean chicken thigh fillets, fat trimmed
- 500ml (2 cups) Massel salt reduced chicken style liquid stock
- 250g cherry tomatoes, halved
- 1 bunch broccolini, cut into 4cm lengths
- 150g snow peas, thinly sliced
- 1 bunch baby buk choy, cut into 4cm lengths
- 1 tablespoon fresh lime juice
- Fresh Thai basil leaves, to serve

METHOD

Step 1: Place noodles in a large heatproof bowl. Cover with boiling water. Set aside for 5 minutes to soften. Drain.

Step 2: Heat oil in a large saucepan over medium heat. Cook onion and celery, stirring, for 5-6 minutes or until softened. Add garlic, ginger, chilli and lemongrass. Cook, stirring, for 1 minute or until aromatic. Add chicken. Cook for 1 minute or until starting to colour.

Step 3: Pour in stock and 750ml (3 cups) water. Bring to the boil. Reduce heat to low. Simmer, partially covered, for 10 minutes or until chicken is cooked through. Remove chicken with tongs. Transfer to a clean board. Set aside to cool slightly. Shred. Return to pan.

Step 4: Add tomato, broccolini and snow peas to soup. Simmer for 3-4 minutes or until vegetables are just tender. Stir through buk choy until just wilted. Stir in lime juice and season. Divide noodles among bowls. Ladle over soup. Serve with basil.

SWEET POTATO SOUP WITH CHORIZO CROUTONS

INGREDIENTS

- 1 tbs olive oil
- 1 brown onion, coarsely chopped
- 600g Kent pumpkin, peeled, seeded, chopped
- 1 gold sweet potato, peeled, chopped
- 4 cups (1L) salt-reduced chicken stock
- 2 Coles Mild Chorizo Salami, chopped
- 3/4 cup (185ml) thickened cream
- 2 tbs pepitas (pumpkin seeds), toasted
- 1/3 cup coriander sprigs

METHOD

Step 1: Heat the oil in a large saucepan over medium heat. Add the onion and cook, stirring, for 2 mins or until onion softens. Add the pumpkin, sweet potato and stock. Bring to the boil. Reduce heat to medium and cook, stirring occasionally, for 20 mins or until the pumpkin is tender. Set aside to cool slightly.

Step 2: Meanwhile, heat a frying pan over high heat. Add chorizo. Cook, stirring, for 5 mins or until golden brown. Transfer to a plate lined with paper towel.

Step 3: Use a stick blender to blend the pumpkin mixture in the saucepan until smooth. Add 1/2 cup (125ml) of the cream and stir to combine. Season.

Step 4: Divide the soup among serving bowls. Drizzle with the remaining cream. Sprinkle with the chorizo, pumpkin seeds and coriander. Season. Serve with the bread.

CHINESE-STYLE LONG AND SHORT SOUP

INGREDIENTS

- 2 tsp sesame oil
- 500g frozen prawn dumplings or pork dumplings
- 4 cups (1L) reduced-salt chicken stock
- 2 tbs reduced-salt soy sauce
- 1 tbs brown sugar
- 5cm-piece ginger, peeled, cut into matchsticks
- 2 garlic cloves, crushed
- 2 cinnamon sticks or quills
- 2 whole star anise
- 2 strips orange rind
- 1 Coles RSPCA Approved Australian Chicken Breast Fillet
- 90g soba noodles
- 1 bunch baby buk choy, quartered lengthways
- 1 tbs chilli oil or sambal oelek (optional)
- 2 spring onions, thinly sliced diagonally

METHOD

Step 1: Heat half the sesame oil in a large saucepan over high heat. Add the dumplings and cook for 2 mins or until golden underneath. Transfer to a plate.

Step 2: Add stock, soy sauce, sugar, ginger, garlic, cinnamon, star anise, orange rind and 2 cups (500ml) water to pan. Bring to the boil. Reduce heat to low. Add the chicken. Cook for 15 mins or until cooked through. Transfer the chicken to a plate. Thinly slice the chicken.

Step 3: Return dumplings to pan with soba noodles. Cook for 5 mins or until tender. Stir in buk choy. Divide among serving bowls. Drizzle with remaining sesame oil. Top with chicken, chilli oil or sambal oelek, if using, and spring onion.

THAI CHICKEN AND RAMEN NOODLE SOUP

INGREDIENTS

- 1/4 cup (75g) yellow or red curry paste
- 4 cups (1L) chicken stock
- 400ml can coconut milk
- 2 Coles RSPCA Approved Australian Chicken Breast Fillets
- 180g ramen noodles
- 125g baby corn, halved lengthways
- 1 tbs lime juice
- 1 tbs brown sugar
- 2 tsp fish sauce
- 1 carrot, peeled, cut into long matchsticks
- 100g snow peas, trimmed, thinly sliced lengthways
- 4 spring onions, cut into long matchsticks

METHOD

Step 1: Heat a large saucepan over high heat. Add the curry paste.

Cook, stirring, for 30 secs or until aromatic. Add the stock and coconut milk and bring to a simmer. Reduce heat to medium-low.

Step 2: Add the chicken to the pan. Cook, turning occasionally, for 15 mins or until chicken is just cooked through. Use a slotted spoon to transfer the chicken to a heatproof bowl. Set aside for 10 mins to cool slightly.

Step 3: Use 2 forks to coarsely shred the chicken. Return to the pan with noodles and corn. Bring to a simmer. Cook for 5 mins or until noodles and corn are tender. Remove from heat. Add lime juice, sugar and fish sauce. Season. Divide among serving bowls. Top with carrot, snow pea and spring onion.

SPEEDY CHICKEN AND EGG NOODLE SOUP

INGREDIENTS

- 4 cups (1L) Salt Reduced Chicken Stock
- 2 spring onions, thinly sliced
- 300g egg noodles
- 1 bunch baby broccoli, halved lengthways
- 1/4 cup (80g) miso paste
- 2 cups shredded Coles Portuguese Hot Roast Chicken
- 3 tsp extra virgin olive oil
- 4 Coles Australian Free Range Eggs
- 3 tsp chilli paste (optional)

METHOD

Step 1: Place the stock and 4 cups (1L) water in a large saucepan over high heat. Bring to the boil. Add half the spring onion to the pan and cook for 2 mins or until aromatic. Add noodles and baby broccoli.

Cook for 3 mins or until noodles are tender. Reduce heat to low. Add the miso and chicken. Stir until combined and heated through.

Step 2: Meanwhile, heat the oil in a large frying pan over high heat. Crack 2 eggs into the pan. Cook for 2 mins or until eggs are golden underneath and the yolks are set or until cooked to your liking. Transfer to a plate. Repeat with the remaining eggs.

Step 3: Divide the noodle mixture evenly among serving bowls. Top with the eggs. Sprinkle with remaining spring onion and drizzle with the chilli paste, if using.

SLOW-COOKED FREEKEH AND LAMB SOUP

INGREDIENTS

- 2 tsp extra virgin olive oil
- 400g lean lamb leg steaks, excess fat trimmed, cut into 1.5cm pieces
- 1 large brown onion, finely chopped
- 2 carrots, peeled, finely chopped
- 3 celery sticks, finely chopped
- 3 garlic cloves, thinly sliced
- 2 tsp finely grated lemon rind
- 1 tsp dried oregano leaves
- 500ml (2 cups) Massel Salt Reduced Chicken Style Liquid Stock
- 100g (1/2 cup) wholegrain freekeh, rinsed, drained
- 200g green beans, sliced
- 150g (1 cup) frozen peas
- 90g (1/3 cup) natural yoghurt
- 2 tbs chopped fresh mint leaves, plus extra sprigs, to serve

METHOD

Step 1: Heat half the oil in a large saucepan over medium-high heat. Cook the lamb, in batches, turning, for 3-4 minutes or until browned. Transfer to a plate.

Step 2: Reduce heat to medium and heat the remaining oil in the pan. Add the onion, carrot and celery. Cook, stirring often, for 5 minutes or until soft. Add garlic, lemon rind and oregano. Cook, stirring, for 1 minute or until aromatic. Return the lamb to the pan along with the stock and 875ml (31 /2 cups) water. Bring to the boil. Add freekeh then reduce heat and simmer, covered, for 11/2-2 hours or until lamb is tender.

Step 3: Add the beans and peas. Simmer, uncovered, for 10 minutes or until the vegetables are tender.

Step 4: Meanwhile, combine the yoghurt and mint in a small bowl.

Step 5: Dollop mint yoghurt onto soup, season and serve with extra mint.

PRAWN AND POTATO SOUP WITH CHILLI TOAST

INGREDIENTS

- 2 tbs olive oil
- 1 brown onion, coarsely chopped
- 50g streaky bacon rashers, finely chopped
- 3 garlic cloves, crushed
- 1/4 cup (60ml) sherry (optional)
- 1 tsp smoked paprika
- 500g Red Royale potatoes, cut into 3cm pieces
- 4 cups (1L) salt-reduced chicken stock
- 400g tomato passata
- 1/2 Coles Bakery Stone Baked by Laurent Sourdough Baguette*, thinly sliced diagonally
- 1 garlic clove, extra, halved
- Tabasco sauce, to serve
- 600g raw prawns, peeled leaving tails intact, deveined
- 2 tbs coarsely chopped flat-leaf parsley

METHOD

Step 1: Preheat oven to 200°C. Line a baking tray with baking paper. Heat half the oil in a large saucepan over medium heat. Add the onion, bacon and crushed garlic. Cook, stirring occasionally, for 5 mins or until onion softens and the bacon is golden brown.

Step 2: Increase heat to high. Add the sherry, if using, and cook, stirring, for 2-3 mins or until liquid reduces. Add the paprika and potato and cook, stirring constantly, for 1 min or until well combined.

Step 3: Add stock, passata and 1/4 cup (60ml) water to the pan and bring to the boil. Reduce heat to low. Cover and cook for 8 mins or until the potatoes are tender.

Step 4: Meanwhile, lightly spray both sides of baguette slices with olive oil spray. Arrange over lined tray. Bake for 5 mins or until golden. Rub both sides of the bread with cut side of the extra garlic. Drizzle with some of the Tabasco.

Step 5: Heat the remaining oil in a large frying pan over high heat. Season. Add prawns and cook, stirring occasionally, for 2 mins or until prawns curl and are cooked through. Stir in half the parsley.

Step 6: Divide soup among serving bowls. Top with the prawns. Sprinkle with the remaining parsley. Serve with chilli toast.

CREAMY BORLOTTI BEAN AND PASTA SOUP

INGREDIENTS

- 1 tablespoon extra virgin olive oil
- 1 brown onion, finely chopped
- 2 carrots, finely chopped
- 2 garlic cloves, finely chopped
- 1 teaspoon finely chopped fresh rosemary leaves
- 1 litre Massel Vegetable Liquid Stock
- 400g can diced tomatoes
- 200g dried spiral pasta
- 400g can borlotti beans, drained, rinsed
- 1/2 cup thickened cream
- 2 tablespoons shaved parmesan
- 2 tablespoons roughly chopped fresh flat-leaf parsley

METHOD

Step 1: Heat oil in a large saucepan over medium-high heat. Add onion, carrot, garlic and rosemary. Cook, stirring, for 5 minutes or until softened. Add stock and tomatoes. Stir. Bring to the boil. Reduce heat to medium. Cook, covered, for 10 minutes. Remove from heat. Using a stick blender, blend soup until smooth. Season with salt and pepper.

Step 2: Return to the boil over medium-high heat. Stir in pasta. Simmer, covered, stirring often, for 12 to 15 minutes or until pasta is tender. Add beans and 1/2 the cream. Stir to combine.

Step 3: Drizzle soup with remaining cream. Serve topped with parmesan, parsley and pepper.

MATT SINCLAIR'S THAI COCONUT SOUP WITH PRAWNS

INGREDIENTS

- 2 x 400ml cans coconut cream
- 1L salt-reduced chicken stock
- 2 stems lemongrass, halved, bruised
- 2.5cm-piece ginger, peeled, cut into matchsticks
- 2 birdseye chillies, halved lengthways
- 1 bunch coriander, leaves picked, roots reserved and bruised
- 5 kaffir lime leaves
- 1kg raw prawns, peeled leaving tails intact, deveined
- 100g oyster mushrooms, torn, or button mushrooms, quartered
- 2 tbs fish sauce
- 1 tbs lime juice
- Pinch of sugar
- Pinch of salt
- Thinly sliced long red chilli, to serve (optional)

METHOD

Step 1: Bring the coconut cream and stock to the boil in a large saucepan over medium-high heat. Add lemongrass, ginger, birdseye chilli and reserved coriander roots. Tear 4 lime leaves and add to the pan. Reduce heat to low and simmer gently for 10 mins.

Step 2 Add prawns and mushroom to the pan. Simmer for 2-3 mins or until prawns change colour. Remove from heat.

Step 3: Stir in the fish sauce, lime juice, sugar and salt. Taste and add more fish sauce, lime juice, sugar and salt if needed.

Step 4: Finely shred remaining kaffir lime leaf. Remove lemongrass from soup and discard. Divide soup among serving bowls. Sprinkle with shredded lime leaf, coriander leaves and chilli, if using.

RECIPE NOTES

Boost the veg: Add extra veggies to the soup if you want to bulk it up. Anything you have in your crisper would work – think carrots, choy sum, buk choy or other mushrooms.

ROASTED CARROT AND PARSNIP SOUP

INGREDIENTS

- 1 parsnip, washed, trimmed and halved lengthways
- 1 kg carrots, washed, trimmed and halved lengthways
- 2 teaspoons brown sugar
- salt and cracked black pepper
- 2 tablespoons olive oil
- 4 cups (1 litre) Massel chicken style liquid stock or vegetable liquid stock
- 2 tablespoons olive oil, extra
- 1/4 cup sage leaves

METHOD

Step 1: Preheat oven to 180°C. Place parsnip and carrot on a baking tray lined with non-stick baking paper. Sprinkle with brown sugar, salt and pepper and drizzle with the oil.

Step 2: Cook parsnip and carrot for 35 minutes or until soft and golden brown. Remove and allow to cool for 10 minutes, then place in a blender or food processor and blend until smooth.

Step 3: Place the parsnip and carrot puree in a large saucepan and add the stock and 2 cups of water. Bring to a high simmer over medium-low heat and cook for 5 minutes or until heated through.

Step 4: Meanwhile, heat the extra oil in a small non-stick frying pan over medium-high heat. Add the sage leaves and fry until crisp and golden. Remove and place on paper towel.

Step 5: To serve, ladle soup into bowls and top with the sage leaves and cracked black pepper.

RECIPE NOTES

When blending vegetables, add a little extra water if the consistency isn't smooth enough.

THAI CORN SOUP

INGREDIENTS

- 3 teaspoons Thai red curry paste
- 400ml coconut milk
- 1 1/2 cups chicken stock
- 400g can sweet corn kernels
- 310g can creamed corn
- 1 tablespoons coriander, chopped
- 2 tomatoes, chopped
- 3 spring onions, chopped

METHOD

Step 1: Place curry paste in a medium saucepan. Stir on low for 1-2 mins, until fragrant. Add coconut milk and stock and bring to the boil.

Step 2: Stir through sweet corn and creamed corn and simmer for 5 mins. Ladle into bowls and top with tomato, onions and coriander, to serve.

CREAM OF CAULIFLOWER SOUP

INGREDIENTS

- 2 tsp olive oil
- 1 brown onion, halved, finely chopped
- 650g cauliflower, cut into florets
- 2 small (about 250g) sebago (brushed) potatoes, peeled, coarsely chopped
- 625ml (2 1/2 cups) Massel vegetable liquid stock
- 330ml (1 1/3 cups) water
- 80ml (1/3 cup) extra light thickened cream
- Extra light thickened cream, extra, to serve
- Ground black pepper, to taste
- Salt, to season

METHOD

Step 1: Heat the oil in a large saucepan over medium heat. Add the onion and cook, stirring, for 5-6 minutes or until soft.

Step 2: Add the cauliflower, potato, stock and water. Cover and bring to the boil. Reduce heat to medium-low and simmer, partially covered, for 15 minutes or until the cauliflower and potato are tender. Set aside for 5 minutes to cool slightly.

Step 3: Place half the cauliflower mixture in the jug of a blender and blend until smooth. Transfer to a clean saucepan. Repeat with remaining mixture. Add the cream. Place over low heat and cook for 1-2 minutes or until heated through.

Step 4: Ladle soup among serving bowls and drizzle with extra cream. Season with pepper.

LENTIL & CANNELLINI BEAN SOUP

INGREDIENTS

- 1 tsp olive oil
- 2 carrots, peeled, finely chopped
- 1 brown onion, halved, finely chopped
- 1 garlic clove, crushed
- 1L (4 cups) Massel vegetable liquid stock
- 1 x 800g can diced Italian tomatoes
- 2 slices prosciutto
- 1 x 400g can brown lentils, rinsed, drained
- 1 x 400g can cannellini beans, rinsed, drained
- Shaved parmesan, to serve
- Baguette (French breadstick), sliced crossways, to serve

METHOD

Step 1: Heat the oil in a large saucepan over medium-high heat. Add the carrot, onion and garlic and cook, stirring, for 3 minutes or until the onion is soft. Add the stock and tomato and bring to the boil. Reduce heat to low and cook, covered, for 15 minutes or until the mixture thickens slightly.

Step 2: Meanwhile, preheat grill on high. Place the prosciutto on a baking tray. Cook under grill for 2 minutes each side or until crisp. Set aside to cool slightly. Coarsely chop.

Step 3: Add the lentils and cannellini beans to the soup and cook, stir-ring, for 2 minutes or until heated through. Taste and season with salt and pepper.

Step 4: Ladle the soup among serving bowls. Top with prosciutto and parmesan. Serve immediately with bread.

INDIAN SPICED CAULIFLOWER SOUP

INGREDIENTS

- 2 tsp vegetable oil
- 1 brown onion, coarsely chopped
- 2 garlic cloves, crushed
- 1 tbsp finely grated ginger
- 1 large green chilli, seeded, finely chopped
- 2 tbsp mild curry paste
- 1 large cauliflower, cut into florets
- 1 large potato, peeled, coarsely chopped
- 1 litre (4 cups) Massel chicken style liquid stock or vegetable liquid stock
- 250ml Bulla Cooking Cream
- 6 sprigs curry leaves
- 2 tbsp vegetable oil, extra, to shallow fry
- Pappadums, to serve

METHOD

Step 1: Heat the oil in a large frying pan over medium-high heat. Add the onion, garlic, ginger and chilli and cook, stirring, for 5 minutes or until onion softens. Add the curry paste and cook for 1 minute or until aromatic.

Step 2; Add the cauliflower, potato and chicken stock and bring to the boil. Reduce heat to low and simmer, stirring occasionally, for 20 minutes or until potato and cauliflower and tender. Remove from heat. Set aside for 5 minutes to cool slightly.

Step 3: Transfer cauliflower mixture to the jug of a blender and blend until smooth.

Step 4: Return to saucepan. Place over low heat. Add the cooking cream and stir to combine. Cook for 2 minutes or until heated through. Taste and season with salt and pepper.

Step 5: Meanwhile, heat extra oil in a small frying pan over medium heat. Add half the curry leaves and cook for 1 minute or until crisp. Transfer to a plate. Repeat with remaining curry leaves.

Step 6; Ladle soup among serving bowls. Top with curry leaves. Serve immediately with pappadums, if desired.

RECIPE NOTES

If you prefer, you can use curry powder instead, but only use 3 teaspoons-1 tablespoon as it's more intense in flavour.

TO FREEZE: Follow recipe until the end of Step 3. Tranfer to an air-tight container and freeze for up to 3 months. To reheat, defrost and continue from Step 4.

CURRIED VEGETABLE AND BEAN SOUP

INGREDIENTS

- 2 tablespoons olive oil
- 2 cloves garlic, crushed
- 1 medium or 2 baby fennel bulbs, trimmed, quartered, thinly sliced
- 2 leeks, trimmed, washed, thinly sliced
- 2 medium Desiree potatoes, peeled, cut into 2cm pieces
- 2 medium zucchini, thinly sliced
- 2 teaspoons Madras curry powder
- 750ml (3 cups) Massel chicken style liquid stock
- 6 thick slices multi-grain bread
- 1 420g can four bean mix, rinsed, drained

METHOD

Step 1: Heat the olive oil in a large saucepan over medium heat and cook garlic for 30 seconds. Add fennel, leeks, potatoes and zucchini and cook, stirring often, for 6-8 minutes or until vegetables begin to soften. Stir in curry powder and cook, stirring constantly, for 2-3 minutes or until vegetables are evenly coated.

Step 2: Stir in chicken stock, cover and bring to the boil. Reduce heat to medium-low and gently boil, stirring occasionally, for 15 minutes or until potatoes are tender.

Step 3: Meanwhile, toast the bread until golden. Add beans to the soup and cook for 1-2 minutes or until heated through. Serve the soup in bowls with the toast.

RECIPE NOTES

For the kids: Vegetable & cheese soup - leave out the curry powder and serve the soup topped with grated cheddar cheese. Cut toast into fingers. Gourmet tip: Add ground cumin to the soup to taste with the curry powder.

PORK SAUSAGE AND BEAN SOUP

INGREDIENTS

- 1/3 cup olive oil
- 12 (900g) pork and fennel sausages
- 4 leeks, trimmed, halved, washed, sliced
- 5 celery stalks, sliced
- 5 garlic cloves, crushed
- 3 x 400g cans diced tomatoes
- 5 x 420g cans four bean mix, drained, rinsed
- 2 litres Massel chicken style liquid stock
- 500g frozen peas
- 1/2 cup basil pesto
- Shaved parmesan, to serve

METHOD

Step 1: Heat 1 tablespoon oil in a large 12-litre capacity stockpot over medium-high heat. Cook sausages in 2 batches, turning, for 10 minutes or until browned. Transfer to a plate. Slice. Discard oil from pot. Wipe pot clean.

Step 2: Heat remaining oil in pot over medium heat. Add leek, celery and garlic. Cook, stirring occasionally, for 3 minutes. Cover. Cook for 5 minutes or until leek has softened. Add tomatoes, beans, stock, sausage and 2 litres cold water. Increase heat to high. Bring to the boil. Reduce heat to medium. Simmer for 15 minutes, adding peas for the last 2 minutes of cooking. Season with salt and pepper.

Step 3: Ladle soup into bowls. Dollop with pesto and serve topped with parmesan.

CHICKEN AND CORN SOUP

INGREDIENTS

- 20g butter
- 2 garlic cloves, finely chopped
- 5 chicken thigh fillets, trimmed and sliced
- 1 litre Massel chicken style liquid stock
- 2 x 420g cans creamed corn
- 2 x 125g cans corn kernels, drained
- 1 tbsp brown sugar
- 1/4 cup sour cream
- salt and cracked black pepper
- 1/3 cup chopped coriander leaves

METHOD

Step 1: Melt the butter in a large saucepan over medium heat. Add the garlic and cook for 1 minute, then add the chicken and cook for 3-4 minutes. Stir in the stock, creamed corn, corn kernels and sugar. Bring to the boil then simmer for 15 minutes or until the chicken is very tender and you're happy with the consistency.

Step 2: Remove from the heat and stir through the sour cream, salt and pepper. Top with the coriander and serve.

SOUTH INDIAN PUMPKIN & COCONUT SOUP

INGREDIENTS

- 1 x 170g pkt Continental South Indian Curry with Roasted Spices Flavour Base
- 1 kg butternut pumpkin, peeled, deseeded, coarsely chopped
- 750ml (3 cups) water
- 185ml (3/4 cup) coconut cream
- 1 tbsp coconut cream, extra, to serve
- 1 tbsp finely chopped fresh chives

METHOD

Step 1: Combine the flavour base, pumpkin and water in a large saucepan over high heat. Bring to the boil. Reduce heat to medium-low and simmer, uncovered, stirring occasionally, for 15-20 minutes or until the pumpkin is tender. Remove from heat and set aside for 5 minutes to cool slightly.

Step 2: Place the pumpkin mixture in the jug of a blender and blend until smooth. Transfer to a saucepan and add the coconut cream. Place over medium heat and cook, stirring, for 5 minutes or until heated through.

Step 3: Ladle the soup among serving bowls. Drizzle with a little extra coconut cream and sprinkle with chives. Serve immediately.

ROASTED CAPSICUM, TOMATO & CORIANDER SOUP

INGREDIENTS

- 2 tsp olive oil
- 1 onion, finely chopped
- 2 garlic cloves, crushed
- 1 long red chilli, seeds removed, finely chopped
- 2 x 400g cans chopped tomatoes
- 3 roasted red capsicums (about 300g), peeled, roughly chopped (see note)
- 2 cups (500ml) Massel vegetable liquid stock
- 1/3 cup (80g) low-fat yoghurt
- Chopped coriander, to garnish

METHOD

Step 1: Heat oil in a large pan over medium heat. Cook onion, stirring occasionally, for 5 minutes or until soft. Add garlic and chilli, and cook, stirring, for 1 minute. Add tomatoes and capsicum, and stir to combine. Add stock, then bring to the boil. Reduce heat to low and simmer for 10 minutes or until the mixture reduces slightly. Set aside to cool a little, then blend, in batches, until smooth.

Step 2: Return soup to pan over medium heat until heated through. Season to taste with sea salt and freshly ground black pepper. Serve garnished with a dollop of low-fat yoghurt and chopped coriander.

CHICKEN, RISONI AND SPINACH SOUP

INGREDIENTS

- 1 onion, roughly chopped
- 1 stick celery, roughly chopped
- 1 carrot, roughly chopped
- 1 bay leaf
- 6 peppercorns
- 4 cups (1L) Massel chicken style liquid stock
- 3 cups (750ml) water
- 2/3 cup risoni pasta
- 2 single chicken breast fillets, thinly sliced, excess fat trimmed
- 1 1/2 cups baby spinach leaves
- salt and cracked black pepper

METHOD

Step 1: Place the onion, celery, carrot, bay leaf and peppercorns in a large saucepan over medium heat. Add stock and water and bring to

94

the boil. Reduce the heat, cover and simmer for 45 minutes then remove from stovetop and strain, reserving the liquid.

Step 2: Return liquid to the pan over medium heat. Add the risoni and simmer for 4 minutes. Add the chicken and cook for another 3-4 minutes. Add the spinach and cook for another 3-4 minutes or until spinach has wilted.

Step 3: Season with salt and pepper. Ladle soup between serving bowls and serve immediately.

FISH AND NOODLE SOUP

INGREDIENTS

- 3 cups Massel chicken style liquid stock
- 2 tsp salt-reduced soy sauce
- 2 carrots, peeled, cut into thin sticks
- 2 celery sticks, thinly sliced
- 2 zucchini, cut into thin sticks
- 200g Swiss brown mushrooms, sliced
- 3cm piece fresh ginger, peeled, grated
- 200g fresh udon noodles
- 400g firm white fish (see note), cut into short, thick strips
- 150g baby spinach

METHOD

Step 1: Place stock, 3 cups cold water and soy sauce in a large saucepan. Bring to the boil over medium heat. Add carrots, celery, zucchini, mushrooms, ginger and noodles. Simmer, partially covered, for 4 minutes.

Step 2: Add fish and simmer for 2 to 3 minutes or until fish is just cooked through. Add spinach. Cook, stirring, for 1 minute or until leaves are wilted. Season with pepper. Serve.

RECIPE NOTES

Note: Flathead or ling are suitable fish for this recipe.

PUMPKIN AND GNOCCHI SOUP

INGREDIENTS

- 2 tbsp olive oil
- 1 brown onion, finely chopped
- 3 garlic cloves, sliced
- 1kg pumpkin, peeled, seeded, cut into 3cm pieces
- 2 cups Massel vegetable liquid stock
- 100g sliced pancetta, torn (optional for a vegetarian option)
- 2 tbsp torn sage leaves
- 700g pkt ready made gnocchi

EQUIPMENT

Hand held blender or blender

METHOD

Step 1: Heat half the oil in a large saucepan over medium heat. Cook onion and garlic for 5 minutes. Add pumpkin and stock and bring to the boil. Reduce heat and simmer, covered, for 15 minutes or until pumpkin is tender. Using a hand held blender, process soup until smooth. Season.

Step 2: Meanwhile, heat remaining oil in a large frying pan over medium-high heat. Cook pancetta and sage for 4-5 minutes or until crisp.

Step 3: Bring a large saucepan of salted water to the boil. Cook gnocchi for 2 minutes or until tender and they rise to the surface. Drain.

Step 4: Divide soup between serving bowls. Add gnocchi and top with pancetta mixture.

RECIPE NOTES

You can freeze the soup after step 1 for up to 1 month.

VEAL TORTELLINI SOUP

INGREDIENTS

- 4 cups (1 litre) Massel beef style liquid stock
- 700ml tomato passata
- 1/2 teaspoon sugar
- salt and cracked black pepper
- 375g veal tortellini (or beef tortellini)
- Fresh basil, shredded, to serve

METHOD

Step 1: Place the stock, tomato passata, sugar, salt and pepper in a large saucepan over medium heat and bring to a high simmer.

Step 2: Add the tortellini and cook following packet instructions or until al dente.

Step 3: To serve, spoon the tortellini among serving bowls and pour over the soup. Sprinkle with basil and serve immediately.

TOFU NOODLE SOUP

INGREDIENTS

- 4 cups (1L) Coles Japanese Inspired Mushroom & Miso Style Broth
- 270g soba noodles
- 5cm-piece ginger, peeled, cut into matchsticks
- 1 carrot, peeled, cut into matchsticks
- 1 bunch baby choy sum, cut into 5cm lengths
- 200g frozen edamame or broad beans, thawed, peeled
- 200g pkt honey soy tofu, thinly sliced
- 2 spring onions, thinly sliced
- 2 tbs Table of Plenty Asian Black Sesame Dukkah Salad Sprinkles

METHOD

Step 1: Place the broth in a large saucepan over high heat. Bring to the boil. Add the noodles and cook for 3 mins or until the noodles are tender.

Step 2: Add the ginger, carrot, choy sum and edamame or broad beans to the pan. Cook for 1 min or until the carrot is just tender and heated through.

Step 3: Divide soup among serving bowls. Top with the tofu and spring onion. Sprinkle with dukkah to serve.

RECIPE NOTES

SWAP ME: Don't have the miso broth? Use regular stock and add mushrooms with the veggies if you have them.

JUICE RECIPES

GREEN VEGGIE JUICE

INGREDIENTS

- 20g baby spinach leaves
- 1 Granny Smith apple, cored, chopped
- 1 Lebanese cucumber, chopped
- 1 kiwifruit, peeled, chopped
- 1 lime, peeled, chopped
- 1 1/2 cups (375ml) coconut water
- 2 tsp finely grated ginger
- Lime slices, to serve

METHOD

Step 1: Place the spinach, apple, cucumber, kiwifruit, chopped lime, coconut water and ginger in a blender and blend until smooth.

Step 2: Pour the spinach mixture into serving glasses. Top with lime slices and serve immediately.

BERRY AND WATERMELON JUICE

INGREDIENTS

- 1/4 watermelon, peeled, chopped
- 125g raspberries
- 250g strawberries, chopped
- 1 cup crushed ice
- Ice cubes, to serve
- Watermelon wedges, to serve
- Mint sprigs, to serve

METHOD

Step 1: Place the chopped watermelon, raspberries, strawberry and crushed ice in a blender and blend until smooth.

Step 2: Pour the watermelon mixture into serving glasses. Top with ice cubes, watermelon wedges and mint to serve.

JINGLE JUICE

INGREDIENTS

- 2 cups cranberry and pomegranate juice
- 1 tbsp caster sugar
- 1/3 cup orange liqueur
- 750ml bottle sparkling white wine, chilled
- 8 cups ice cubes
- 1 small orange, cut into 8 thin slices
- 2/3 cup frozen pomegranate seeds
- Fresh mint leaves, to serve

METHOD

Step 1: Place juice and sugar in a small saucepan over medium heat. Cook, stirring, for 2 to 3 minutes or until sugar has dissolved. Set aside to cool completely.

Step 2: Combine juice mixture, liqueur and sparkling wine in a large jug. Divide ice cubes and orange slices among 8 x 470ml-capacity glasses. Pour juice mixture into glasses. Top with pomegranate seeds and mint. Serve.

SWAMP JUICE

INGREDIENTS

- 85g packet lime jelly crystals
- 2 cups boiling water
- 1/3 cup glucose syrup
- 2 drops green food colouring
- 1.5 litres chilled pineapple juice

METHOD

Step 1: Place jelly crystals in a large heatproof bowl. Add boiling water. Whisk until crystals have dissolved. Stir in 200ml cold water. Allow to cool for 30 minutes.

Step 2: Place glucose syrup in a small heatproof, microwave-safe bowl. Microwave on HIGH (100%) for 20 seconds or until runny. Tint green with food colouring. Spoon mixture into a snap-lock bag. Snip off one corner. Working quickly, pipe mixture around the inside top of eight 1 cup-capacity glasses. Stand for 1 minute or until mixture starts to run down the inside of each glass. Refrigerate for 5 to 10 minutes or until set.

Step 3: Add pineapple juice to jelly mixture. Stir to combine. Just before serving, divide juice between glasses. Serve immediately.

PEARS POACHED IN CRANBERRY JUICE

INGREDIENTS

- 500mls (2 cups) cranberry juice
- 50g (1/4 cup, firmly packed) brown sugar
- 1 cinnamon stick
- 4 (about 250g each) just ripe pears (like beurre bosc, packham or williams), peeled
- Thick cream or natural yoghurt, to serve

METHOD

Step 1: Combine the cranberry juice, brown sugar and cinnamon stick in a saucepan large enough to hold the pears standing upright. Stir over medium heat until the sugar dissolves. Bring to the boil and reduce heat to medium-low.

Step 2: Add the pears and simmer, uncovered, spooning the juices over and carefully rotating the pears occasionally (this will help them colour evenly), for 40-50 minutes or until tender.

Step 3: Remove from heat and cool pears for 30 minutes in the syrup. Discard cinnamon stick.

Step 4: Serve the pears warm with the cream or yoghurt, or cool completely in the syrup and serve at room temperature.

RECIPE NOTES

Microwave tip: Place cranberry juice, brown sugar and cinnamon stick in a large heat-resistant, microwave-safe bowl. Cook, uncovered, for 3-4 minutes, stirring twice, on High/850watts/100% or until the sugar dissolves. Add the pears and cook, uncovered, for 15-18 minutes on Medium/500watts/50% or until tender.

APPLE, BROCCOLI AND LEMON JUICE

INGREDIENTS

- 4 large granny smith apples, unpeeled, cored, chopped
- 1 cup (85g) broccoli florets
- 1 lemon, skin and rind removed

METHOD

Step 1: Place a jug under juice extractor nozzle. Juice apple, broccoli and lemon. Stir to combine. Pour into chilled glasses. Serve.

APPLE, SPINACH AND MINT JUICE

INGREDIENTS

- 5 green apples
- 4 celery stalks
- 100g baby spinach leaves
- 2 cups mint leaves
- 1 lime, peeled

METHOD

Step 1: Pass all ingredients through a juicer, then transfer to a jug and serve.

SUPER GREEN JUICE

INGREDIENTS

- 1/2 small bunch English spinach, washed, roots trimmed
- 2 green apples, quartered
- 4 stalks fresh mint
- 2 Lebanese cucumbers
- 2 large stalks parsley, optional

METHOD

Step 1: Using a Breville Froojie Fountain juicer, process the spinach, apples, mint, cucumber and parsley.

Step 2: Stir in the Greens Powder if using and pour into glasses to serve.

RECIPE NOTES

For added nutrition, stir in 1 tsp of Greens powder , just before serving.

PINK PEPPERED BERRY JUICE

INGREDIENTS

- 1 (130g) ripe yellow nectarine, skin on, stone removed
- 3-4 large (120 g) strawberries, washed and hulled
- 200 g seedless watermelon flesh
- 1/4 cup frozen raspberries
- 200ml organic apple juice (no added sugar)
- 1 teaspoon crushed pink pepper corns

METHOD

Step 1: Place the nectarine flesh, strawberries, watermelon and raspberries in a Breville Kinetix Control blender. Add the apple juice and half the pepper. Blend for 15-20 seconds or until smooth.

Step 2: Pour into chilled glasses and sprinkle over the remaining pepper.

COCONUT MANGO FROOJIE

INGREDIENTS

- 1 mango, peeled and seed removed
- 1 whole young coconut
- 1 teaspoon ground cardamom
- 1 teaspoon vanilla extract
- 2-3 teaspoons maple syrup or honey, to sweeten, optional
- 1/4 cup oat milk

METHOD

Step 1: Crack the coconut with a large sharp knife or cleaver. Pour the milk into a jug and set aside. Scoop out the soft flesh. Using a Breville Froojie Fountain juicer, process the mango and coconut flesh at low speed into the jug.

Step 2: Add the coconut milk, cardamom, vanilla and maple syrup or honey to the jug. Stir well to combine. Pour into chilled glasses to serve.

PINA COLADA GREEN JUICE

INGREDIENTS

- 1 banana, peeled, chopped
- 1/2 small pineapple, peeled, cored, chopped
- 2 kiwifruit, peeled, coarsely chopped
- 1/2 baby cos lettuce, trimmed, chopped
- 1/2 cup baby spinach
- 3/4 cup fresh mint leaves, chopped
- 250ml (1 cup) apple juice
- 330ml (1 1/3 cups) coconut water
- 1 lime, juiced
- Crushed ice, to serve
- Lime slices, to serve
- Fresh mint sprigs, to serve

METHOD

Step 1: Place banana, pineapple, kiwifruit, lettuce, spinach, mint, apple juice, coconut water and lime juice in a large blender. Blend until smooth.

Step 2: Serve the juice over ice, garnished with lime slices and mint sprigs.

SUMMER PARTY PUNCH

INGREDIENTS

- 1 star anise
- 1/2 cup caster sugar
- 1/3 cup water
- 2 cups pineapple juice
- 1 cup chilled sparkling mineral water
- 125g raspberries
- 120g blueberries
- 100g seedless green grapes, halved
- 100g seedless red grapes, halved
- 1 mango, peeled, sliced
- 2 kiwifruits, peeled, cut into wedges
- 1 small red apple, sliced crossways
- 1/2 cup fresh mint sprigs
- Ice cubes, to serve
- Lemon slices, to serve

METHOD

Step 1: Place star anise, 1/3 cup sugar and 1/3 cup water in a small saucepan. Stir over medium heat for 2 minutes or until sugar dissolves. Remove from heat. Place in a large bowl. Stir in pineapple juice and mineral water.

Step 2: Place fruit, half the mint and ice in a large jug. Top with juice mixture. Serve punch with lemon slices and top with remaining mint.

GREEN POWER SLUSHIE

INGREDIENTS

- 1/4 (450g) pineapple
- 1 cup firmly packed baby spinach
- 1/4 cup firmly packed fresh mint leaves
- 2 tablespoons lemon juice
- 3 cups ice cubes

METHOD

Step 1: Remove and discard skin from pineapple and roughly chop. Place in a blender with the spinach, mint, lemon juice and ice cubes. Blend until smooth.

Step 2: Pour into 2 x chilled 2-cup-capacity glasses. Serve immediately.

ORANGE AND BEETROOT SLUSHIE

INGREDIENTS

- 1 medium (190g) trimmed beetroot
- 2 oranges, peeled, roughly chopped
- 1 cup passionfruit sorbet
- 3 cups ice cubes

METHOD

Step 1: Wearing disposable gloves, peel and cut beetroot into 2cm pieces. Place in a blender with the orange, sorbet and ice cubes. Blend until smooth.

Step 2: Pour into 2 x chilled 2-cup-capacity glasses. Serve immediately.

BERRY AND WATERMELON JUICE

INGREDIENTS

- 1/4 watermelon, peeled, chopped
- 125g raspberries
- 250g strawberries, chopped
- 1 cup crushed ice
- Ice cubes, to serve
- Watermelon wedges, to serve
- Mint sprigs, to serve

EQUIPMENT

Blender

METHOD

Step 1: Place the chopped watermelon, raspberries, strawberry and crushed ice in a blender and blend until smooth.

Step 2: Pour the watermelon mixture into serving glasses. Top with ice cubes, watermelon wedges and mint to serve.

RECIPE NOTES

DIY fruit iceblocks For a cool treat, freeze the watermelon mixture to make iceblocks. Simply divide mixture among moulds, insert iceblock sticks and freeze.

STRAWBERRY, ORANGE & PAPAYA JUICE

INGREDIENTS

- 8 oranges, peeled, white pith removed
- 500g (2 punnets) strawberries, washed, hulled
- 400g red papaya, skin removed, deseeded, cut into chunks

METHOD

Step 1: Push the oranges, strawberries and papaya through the feed tube of a juicer. Serve immediately.

ECHINACEA AND VEGETABLE JUICE

INGREDIENTS

- 1 echinacea tea bag
- 80ml (1/3 cup) boiling water
- 2 large carrots, peeled, topped
- 1 red capsicum, halved, deseeded, thickly sliced
- 1 lime, peeled
- Ice cubes (optional), to serve

METHOD

Step 1: Place the tea bag in a small heatproof bowl and pour over boiling water. Set aside for 10 minutes to infuse.

Step 2: Meanwhile, use a juice extractor to process the carrot, capsicum and lime. Transfer to a small jug. Squeeze all the liquid from the tea bag. Pour the tea into the jug. Add the ice cubes and stir to combine. Pour among glasses to serve.

CHAMPAGNE AND POMEGRANATE JUICE

INGREDIENTS

- 300ml pomegranate juice (or cranberry)
- 750ml Champagne or sparkling wine
- Middle Eastern pickled vegetables (see note), to serve

METHOD

Step 1: Divide juice among glasses and top with wine. Serve with pickled vegetables.

APRICOT CRANBERRY BELLINIS

INGREDIENTS

- 1/2 cup apricot nectar
- 1 1/2 cups cranberry juice
- Champagne
- Fresh cherries, to garnish
- Mint leaves, to garnish
- Coles bakery croissants, to serve
- Butter, to serve
- Jam, to serve

METHOD

Step 1: Divide apricot nectar between 6 x 3/4-cup capacity glasses. Add cranberry juice.

Step 2: Top up glasses with champagne, and add a few cherries to each glass. Garnish with mint leaves and serve immediately with croissants, butter and jam.

APPLE, CAMPARI AND MINT PUNCH

INGREDIENTS

- 1 litre Coles apple juice
- 3 cups Coles natural sparkling mineral water
- 1 cup campari
- 1 cup mint leaves
- 2 red apples, thinly sliced
- 4 cups crushed ice

METHOD

Step 1: Combine all ingredients in a large jug. Pour into martini glasses and serve.

GREEN SMOOTHIES

INGREDIENTS

- 3 kale leaves, centre stem removed
- 1 Lebanese cucumber, coarsely chopped
- 1 lime, peeled, coarsely chopped
- 1 green apple, cored, coarsely chopped
- 2cm-piece fresh ginger, peeled, chopped
- 1 mint sprig
- 1 1/2 cups (375ml) no-added-sugar coconut water
- Mint sprigs, extra, to serve
- Lime wedges, to serve

METHOD

Step 1: Place kale, cucumber, lime, apple, ginger, mint and coconut water in a blender and blend until very smooth.

Step 2: Divide between serving glasses. Serve immediately with extra mint and lime.

CITRUS CIRCUS JUICE

INGREDIENTS

- 1 large ruby grapefruit, peeled, quartered
- 2 lemons, peeled, quartered
- 2 mandarins, peeled, segmented
- 4 oranges, peeled, quartered
- 1 lime, peeled, quartered

EQUIPMENT

blender

METHOD

Step 1: Place all ingredients in a blender or juicer. Blend until smooth.

Step 2: Pour into glasses. Serve.

FRESH PINK LEMONADE

INGREDIENTS

- 1 1/2 cups (375ml) lemon juice
- 1 cup (220g) caster sugar
- 3 cups (750ml) water
- 1 lemon, sliced, to garnish
- Fresh mint leaves, to garnish
- RASPBERRY PUREE
- 50g fresh raspberries or frozen raspberries
- 1 tbsp caster sugar, extra
- 1 lemon, sliced

METHOD

Step 1: Stir lemon juice, caster sugar and water in a saucepan over low heat for 5 mins or until sugar dissolves. Cool, then chill for 1 hour.

Step 2: Meanwhile prepare the raspbeery puree: Combine raspberries and extra caster sugar in a saucepan over low heat. Cook, stirring to lightly crush, for 2 mins or until sugar dissolves and raspberries break down and release their juices. Strain through a fine sieve into a bowl.

Step 3: Place the lemonade in a serving jug. Add 1 tablespoon of the raspberry puree and stir to combine. Add sliced lemon, mint leaves and ice cubes to the lemonade. Divide remaining raspberry puree among serving glasses. Top with the pink lemonade.

PASSIONFRUIT PUNCH

INGREDIENTS

- 2 cups orange juice
- 2 cups pineapple juice
- 2 cups lemonade
- 6 passionfruit

METHOD

Step 1: Pour half the orange juice into ice-cube trays and freeze overnight.

Step 2: Cut passionfruit in half and scoop out pulp with a teaspoon. Combine with juices and lemonade in a jug. Serve over orange-juice ice-cubes.

POWER PUNCH JUICE

INGREDIENTS

- 2 stalks kale
- 1/2 medium beetroot, trimmed, peeled
- 2cm-piece fresh ginger
- 1 carrot, peeled, quartered
- 2 celery stalks, trimmed, chopped
- 2 small lemons, peeled, quartered
- 1 1/2 cups water, iced

EQUIPMENT

blender

METHOD

Step 1: Remove and discard stems from kale. Roughly chop leaves.

Step 2: Place all ingredients in a blender. Blend until smooth. Pour into glasses. Serve.

RECIPE NOTES

This drink is best made using chilled fresh ingredients. Alternatively, add ice when blending or serve drinks over ice cubes.

PINEAPPLE, ORANGE AND PASSIONFRUIT SLUSHY

INGREDIENTS

- 4 passionfruit
- 2 cups pineapple juice
- 4 oranges, juiced (to make 2 cups)
- 2 cups crushed ice
- 1/4 cup mint leaves, plus extra to serve

METHOD

Step 1: Strain passionfruit pulp into a jug. Reserve seeds.

Step 2: Combine pineapple orange, passionfruit juice, ice and mint in a food processor or blender. Blend until smooth. Stir through passionfruit seeds.

Step 3: Pour into glasses and garnish with mint leaves.

LYCHEE FLING

INGREDIENTS

- 2 cups ice cubes, crushed
- 185g (1 cup) canned lychees, drained reserving syrup, halved
- 125ml (1/2 cup) reserved lychee syrup
- 50ml Galliano Vanilla liqueur
- 30ml Cointreau liqueur
- 30ml vanilla vodka
- 1/4 cup fresh mint leaves
- 180ml (3/4 cup) pineapple juice, chilled
- Fresh mint leaves, extra, to serve

METHOD

Step 1: Divide the ice between two 450ml glasses. Add the lychees and syrup. Pour over the Galliano, Cointreau and vodka. Add the mint and stir to combine. Top with pineapple juice and extra mint.

ORANGE, VANILLA AND STRAWBERRY JUICE

INGREDIENTS

- 5 oranges, peeled
- 250g punnet strawberries
- Juice of 1/2 lemon
- 1 teaspoon vanilla extract

METHOD

Step 1: Pass the oranges and strawberries through a juicer, then transfer to a jug.

Step 2: Stir through the lemon juice and vanilla.

SPARKLING ELDERFLOWER AND RASPBERRY COCKTAIL

INGREDIENTS

- 2/3 cup (165ml) elderflower cordial
- 750ml bottle sparkling wine, chilled
- Raspberries, to serve

METHOD

Step 1: Pour 2 tablespoons elderflower cordial into each of 6 champagne flutes. Top up with chilled sparkling wine, then serve each cocktail garnished with raspberries.

MORNING BURST

INGREDIENTS

- 3 cups cranberry juice, chilled
- 2 large carrots, chopped
- 2 large oranges, peeled, halved
- 2cm piece fresh ginger, peeled

EQUIPMENT

You'll need a juice extractor.

METHOD

Step 1: Divide cranberry juice between chilled glasses.

Step 2: Place a large jug under juice extractor nozzle. Juice carrot, orange and ginger. Stir to combine.

Step 3: Gently pour one-quarter carrot juice mixture, over the back of a spoon, over cranberry juice in 1 glass to create layers. Repeat with remaining carrot juice mixture. Serve.

APPLE, PEAR AND SPINACH JUICE

INGREDIENTS

- 3 large packham pears, quartered
- 3 large granny smith apples, quartered
- 100g baby spinach
- 5 fresh mint sprigs
- Ice cubes, to serve
- Mint sprigs, to serve

EQUIPMENT

You'll need a juice extractor.

METHOD

Step 1: Place a large jug under juice extractor nozzle. Juice pear, apple, spinach and mint. Stir to combine.

Step 2: Divide ice cubes between chilled glasses. Top with pear juice mixture. Serve with mint.

FRUITY CLEANSER

INGREDIENTS

- Flesh of 1/4 Seedless Watermelon
- 1/2 cup (125ml) grape juice
- 1 cup (250ml) cranberry juice

METHOD

Step 1: Process watermelon in a juicer. Place watermelon juice in a jug with remaining ingredients and stir well to combine. Serve over ice.

SPICED APPLE JUICE

INGREDIENTS

- 2L (8 cups) apple juice
- 2 x 7cm cinnamon sticks, lightly crushed
- 6 whole cloves
- 4 strips orange peel
- 4 strips lemon peel
- 2 granny smith apples, peeled, cored, thinly sliced
- Ice cubes, to serve

METHOD

Step 1: Place the apple juice, cinnamon, cloves and combined peel in a saucepan over high heat. Bring to the boil. Reduce heat to low and simmer for 5 minutes or until aromatic. Set aside for 10 minutes to cool. Transfer to an airtight container and place in the fridge for 2 hours to chill.

Step 2: Strain the juice into a jug. Divide the apple and ice among serving glasses. Pour over the juice and serve.

RECIPE NOTES

Prep: 5 mins (+ 10 mins cooling & 2 hours chilling time) Carry out step 1 up to 1 day ahead. Store in an airtight container in the fridge. Continue from step 2 just before serving.

FRESH WATERMELON JUICE

INGREDIENTS

- 1/2 (about 2.2kg) seedless watermelon, peeled, coarsely chopped
- 2 tsp finely grated ginger
- 2 tbsp lemon juice
- Mint leaves, to serve
- Ice cubes, to serve

METHOD

Step 1: Place watermelon, ginger and lemon juice in the jug of a blender and blend until smooth. Add sugar, if desired.

Step 2: Strain through a fine sieve into a serving jug. Add mint and ice cubes and stir to combine. Serve immediately.

CELERY, APPLE AND GINGER JUICE

INGREDIENTS

- 6 sticks celery, trimmed
- 6 granny smith apples, cut in half, each half cut into wedges
- 5cm-piece fresh ginger, peeled, sliced

METHOD

Step 1: Use a juice extractor to process the celery, apples and ginger. Transfer to a large jug and stir to combine. Serve immediately.

HOT SPICED APPLE JUICE

INGREDIENTS

- 4 apples
- 2 cinnamon sticks
- 4 cardamom pods, cracked

METHOD

Step 1: Remove cores from apples. Cut apples into 2cm cubes.

Step 2: Place apple, cinnamon and cardamom in a large saucepan. Pour over 5 cups cold water. Place over medium heat and bring to the boil.

Step 3: Reduce heat to low. Simmer, partially covered, for 18 to 20 minutes or until apple is soft.

Step 4: Strain juice into a jug. Pour into heatproof glasses and serve.

RECIPE NOTES

Tip: This juice can be stored in an airtight container in the fridge for up to 2 days. To reheat, pour into individual cups and microwave on HIGH (100%) for 1-minute or until hot.

CARROT, BEETROOT, APPLE AND CELERY JUICE

INGREDIENTS

- 2 carrots
- 1 small beetroot
- 2 apples
- 1 celery stick
- 2 oranges, peeled
- 1cm slice of ginger

METHOD

Step 1: Chill ingredients.

Step 2: Feed the vegetables and fruit through a juice maker. Pour juice over crushed ice and serve immediately.

HOMEMADE CITRUSADE

INGREDIENTS

- 1 1/2 cups (375ml) fresh orange juice
- 1 1/2 cups (375ml) fresh pink grapefruit juice
- 1/2 cup (125ml) fresh lemon juice
- 2/3 cup (150g) caster sugar
- Ice cubes, to serve
- Mint leaves, to serve
- Orange slices, to serve
- Lemon slices, to serve
- 1L (4 cups) sparkling mineral water

METHOD

Step 1: Stir fruit juices and sugar together in a large jug until sugar dissolves.

Step 2: Add ice, mint, and orange and lemon slices, then top with mineral water.

GIN AND JUICE

INGREDIENTS

- 120ml Tanqueray Gin
- 360ml freshly squeezed ruby grapefruit juice
- 1 ruby grapefruit, sliced into wheels or slices
- Ice cubes

METHOD

Step 1: Fill a jug with ice then pour in gin.

Step 2: Top with freshly squeezed grapefruit juice then stir well.

Step 3: Garnish with grapefruit wheels then serve.

ORANGE BOOST JUICE

INGREDIENTS

- 2 oranges, peeled, chopped
- 2 carrots, chopped
- 1 mango, peeled, seeded, chopped
- Ice cubes, to serve

METHOD

Step 1: Using a juice extractor, process the orange, carrot and mango.

Step 2: Serve over ice.

ORANGE, CARROT AND CORIANDER REFRESHER

INGREDIENTS

- 3 oranges, peeled
- 2 large carrots
- 1 green apple, quartered
- 2 coriander sprigs with roots, washed

METHOD

Step 1: Using a Breville Froojie Fountain juicer, process the oranges, carrots, apple and coriander.

Step 2: Pour into glasses to serve.

PINEAPPLE, CUCUMBER, BABY COS AND MINT COOLER

INGREDIENTS

- 1/4 sweet pineapple (select a Bethonga , Sweet Gold or similar variety)
- 1 Lebanese cucumber
- 1 green apple, quartered
- 3 stalks fresh mint
- 1 baby cos lettuce, quartered

METHOD

Step 1: Cut the skin from the pineapple and discard. Using a Breville Froojie Fountain juicer, process pineapple, cucumber, apple, mint and baby cos lettuce.

Step 2: Pour into glasses to serve.

PINK PEPPERED BERRY JUICE

INGREDIENTS

- 1 (130g) ripe yellow nectarine, skin on, stone removed
- 3-4 large (120 g) strawberries, washed and hulled
- 200 g seedless watermelon flesh
- 1/4 cup frozen raspberries
- 200ml organic apple juice (no added sugar)
- 1 teaspoon crushed pink pepper corns

METHOD

Step 1: Place the nectarine flesh, strawberries, watermelon and raspberries in a Breville Kinetix Control blender. Add the apple juice and half the pepper. Blend for 15-20 seconds or until smooth.

Step 2: Pour into chilled glasses and sprinkle over the remaining pepper.

APPLE, SPINACH AND MINT JUICE

INGREDIENTS

- 5 green apples
- 4 celery stalks
- 100g baby spinach leaves
- 2 cups mint leaves
- 1 lime, peeled

METHOD

Step 1: Pass all ingredients through a juicer, then transfer to a jug and serve.

DETOX SUPPORT JUICE

INGREDIENTS

- 4 large carrots, unpeeled, ends trimmed
- 4 celery sticks, leaves attached, washed
- 1/2 beetroot, scrubbed
- 6 sprigs fresh continental parsley
- 4cm-piece fresh ginger, washed, unpeeled
- Ice cubes, to serve

METHOD

Step 1: Cut the vegetables into large pieces. Use a juice extractor to process the carrot, celery, beetroot, parsley and ginger into a jug. Pour among glasses. Serve with ice, if desired.

PROSECCO WITH BLOOD ORANGE JUICE

INGREDIENTS

- Blood oranges
- Italian prosecco or spumante (sparkling white wine)

Step 1: Half fill a Champagne or cocktail glass with freshly squeezed blood orange juice, then top up with chilled Italian prosecco or spumante (sparkling white wine).

MANGO SORBET IN SPARKLING APPLE JUICE

INGREDIENTS

- 400g frozen mango dessert (Weis Frutia brand)
- 375ml (1 1/2 cups) chilled sparkling apple juice

METHOD

Step 1: Place 3 scoops of frozen mango dessert in each serving glass. Pour over the sparkling apple juice and serve.

RECIPE NOTES

You can substitute chilled sparkling white wine for the apple juice, if desired. Leftovers: Use the frozen mango dessert in fruit juice smoothies.

WARM APPLE JUICE WITH GINGER AND CINNAMON

INGREDIENTS

- 2L bottled apple juice
- Strips of lemon rind from 1 lemon
- 2cm piece ginger, finely sliced
- 8 cinnamon sticks
- 1 green apple, thinly sliced

METHOD

Step 1: Place apple juice in a jug with lemon rind, ginger and 2 cinnamon sticks. Leave to infuse for 1 hour, then transfer to a saucepan. Heat gently and strain into heatproof glasses. Place a cinnamon stick and an apple slice into each glass, and serve warm.

GREEN POWER SLUSHIE

INGREDIENTS

- 1/4 (450g) pineapple
- 1 cup firmly packed baby spinach
- 1/4 cup firmly packed fresh mint leaves
- 2 tablespoons lemon juice
- 3 cups ice cubes

METHOD

Step 1: Remove and discard skin from pineapple and roughly chop. Place in a blender with the spinach, mint, lemon juice and ice cubes. Blend until smooth.

SPICED APPLE JUICE

INGREDIENTS

- 2L (8 cups) apple juice
- 2 x 7cm cinnamon sticks, lightly crushed
- 6 whole cloves
- 4 strips orange peel
- 4 strips lemon peel
- 2 granny smith apples, peeled, cored, thinly sliced
- Ice cubes, to serve

METHOD

Step 1: Place the apple juice, cinnamon, cloves and combined peel in a saucepan over high heat. Bring to the boil. Reduce heat to low and simmer for 5 minutes or until aromatic. Set aside for 10 minutes to cool. Transfer to an airtight container and place in the fridge for 2 hours to chill.

Step 2: Strain the juice into a jug. Divide the apple and ice among serving glasses. Pour over the juice and serve.

PINK DRINK

INGREDIENTS

- 2 red apples, cut into wedges, core removed
- 1 pink grapefruit, peeled, segmented
- 1 x 250g punnet strawberries, hulled, washed

METHOD

Step 1: Use a juice extractor to process the apple and grapefruit. Transfer to the jug of a blender. Add the strawberries and blend until smooth.

Step 2: Pour among serving glasses and serve immediately.

SPACE PUNCH

INGREDIENTS

- 4 cups (1 litre) pineapple juice, chilled
- 3 cups soda water, chilled
- 1 large apple
- 700g seedless watermelon

METHOD

Step 1: Combine pineapple juice and soda water in a jug or punch bowl.

Step 2: Cut apple lengthways into 1cm-thick slices. Using a 4cm star-shaped cookie cutter, cut stars from apple slices. Using a melon baller, scoop balls from watermelon.

Step 3: Add melon planets and apple stars to the juice mixture. Serve.

COSMOPOLITAN

INGREDIENTS

- 45ml Smirnoff Red Vodka
- 15ml Triple sec liqueur
- 10ml freshly squeezed lime juice
- 30ml cranberry juice
- Orange zest, julienned or lime wedge, to garnish
- cubed ice

METHOD

Step 1: Combine all ingredients in a cocktail shaker or mason jar.

Step 2: Add cubed ice and shake for 10 - 15 seconds.

Step 3: Strain into martini glass.

Step 4: Garnish with finely julienned orange zest or a lime wedge.

LIME AND GINGER SLUSHIE

INGREDIENTS

- 1/4 cup (60ml) lime juice
- 1 1/2 cups (375ml) ginger beer

METHOD

Step 1: Combine the lime juice and ginger beer and pour into a non-metallic tray. Cover and place in the freezer for 1 hour.

Step 2: Remove from the freezer and using a fork, break up the ice crystals. Return to the freezer for another 30 minutes then remove and break up the ice crystals with a fork again. Spoon mixture into small serving glasses and serve immediately.

LEMON-LIME FIZZ

INGREDIENTS

- 160ml lime juice cordial
- 1 1/4 litre lemonade
- 500ml lemon sorbet
- Lemon slices or lime slices, to serve

METHOD

Step 1: Place 1 tablespoon lime cordial into each glass (1 cup capacity). Divide the lemonade between the glasses then add a scoop of sorbet. Add lemon and/or lime slices and serve immediately.

RASPBERRY FIZZ

INGREDIENTS

- 1/2 cup (75g) frozen raspberries
- 1 tablespoon caster sugar
- 2 teaspoons lemon juice
- Fresh raspberries, to serve
- 750ml btl chilled sparkling wine (see tip)
- Mint leaves, to serve

METHOD

Step 1: Combine frozen raspberries, sugar and lemon juice in a saucepan over medium heat. Cook, stirring, for 5 mins or until raspberries break down and release their juices. Remove from heat. Strain through a fine sieve into a jug, using the back of a spoon to press as much liquid through as possible. Discard solids. Place in fridge for 30 mins to chill.

Step 2: Thread fresh raspberries onto skewers. Pour raspberry mixture evenly among serving glasses. Top with wine, raspberry skewers and mint leaves.

WHISKY SPRITZ

INGREDIENTS

- 30ml Johnnie Walker Red Label Scotch Whisky
- 60ml dry ginger ale
- 90ml sparkling apple juice
- 1 lemon wedge
- Ice

METHOD

Step 1: Fill a tall glass with ice.

Step 2: Add 30ml Johnnie Walker scotch whisky.

Step 3: Pour in dry ginger ale, then gently squeeze a wedge of lemon before dropping it in the glass as garnish.

Step 4: Top with sparkling apple juice and stir.

YOUNG COCONUT & BERRY SLUSHIES

INGREDIENTS

- 6 x 300ml plastic cups young coconut juice
- 1/3 cup (50g) frozen raspberries, plus extra raspberries to garnish

METHOD

Step 1: Tip coconut juice and flesh into a blender with berries. Blend until almost smooth, then return to containers and seal with lids.

Step 2: Freeze for at least 4 hours or overnight. Remove from the freezer 2 hours before serving – the juice will thaw into a soft 'slushie'.

Step 3: To serve, top each cup with the remaining berries and tuck in straws and a spoon.

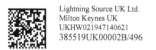
Lightning Source UK Ltd.
Milton Keynes UK
UKHW021947140621
385519UK00002B/496